ZERO POINT WEIGHT LOSS COOKBOOK FOR BEGINNERS

Simple, Delicious, and Guilt-Free Recipes to Lose Weight Without Counting Calories or Stress

Copyright and Disclaimer for "ZERO POINT WEIGHT LOSS COOKBOOK FOR BEGINNERS"

Simple, Delicious, and Guilt-Free Recipes to Lose Weight Without Counting Calories or Stress

By Jean Brown

Table of Content

Introduction

Are you tired of counting every calorie, calculating points, or feeling guilty every time you enjoy a meal? Let's face it, losing weight can feel like a never-ending battle. You've probably tried countless diets, each promising miraculous results, only to find yourself counting every calorie and stressing over every meal. Enter the Zero Point Approach—a fresh, simple, and effective way to enjoy food without the usual hassle of calorie counting. The struggle to find a sustainable, enjoyable way to shed pounds without sacrificing the joy of eating is real.

"ZERO POINT WEIGHT LOSS COOKBOOK FOR BEGINNERS"

Simple, Delicious, and Guilt-Free Recipes to Lose Weight Without Counting Calories or Stress is designed to take the stress out of meal planning and introduce you to a world where delicious, guilt-free eating is possible. It is based on Weight Watchers' ZeroPoint foods list, a revolutionary approach that allows you to enjoy certain foods without the need to track or measure every bite.

Why ZeroPoint foods? The concept is simple: these foods are nutritious, satisfying, and naturally low in calories. They include everyday essentials like fruits, vegetables, lean proteins, and whole grains. By focusing on these foods, you can create meals that are both filling and weight-friendly. This approach is perfect for those who want to eat mindfully without the hassle of constant tracking.

Throughout this book, you'll discover how the ZeroPoint approach is uniquely suited for those seeking a balanced lifestyle. It's not about restriction; it's about abundance. You'll learn how to fill your plate with a variety of flavors and textures, ensuring every meal is a delight. The recipes are crafted to be simple and accessible, making it easy for anyone, regardless of cooking experience, to whip up something tasty and healthy.

You'll learn what makes the ZeroPoint approach stand out, including its emphasis on whole foods and flexibility. We'll also share must-have tools for efficient cooking, ensuring your kitchen is equipped for success. Shopping tips and strategies will help you fill your pantry with the ingredients you need to create satisfying meals without breaking the bank.

Each chapter is dedicated to a different category, from breakfast to dessert. You'll find everything you need to start your day off right, satisfy your snack cravings, and impress at dinner parties. Whether you're in the mood for a hearty stew, a fresh salad, or a sweet treat, there's something here for everyone.

To make your journey even easier, we've included a 30-day meal plan. This plan offers a roadmap to integrating ZeroPoint meals into your daily routine, helping you make lasting changes without the stress of weekly planning. And for those who love to explore, the full ZeroPoint foods list at the end of the book provides endless inspiration for creating your own culinary masterpieces.

"Zero Point Weight Loss Cookbook for Beginners" is more than just a collection of recipes; it's a guide to a healthier, happier you. Let's embark on this journey together, embracing a lifestyle where you can enjoy food without the guilt. Your path to delicious, stress-free eating starts here.

CHAPTER 1

What is the Zero Point Approach?

The Zero Point Approach is a system developed by Weight Watchers that assigns a point value to foods based on their nutritional content. Some foods are classified as "Zero Point" foods because they are low in calories and high in nutrients1. This means you can eat these foods without worrying about adding to your daily points allowance. It's a win-win situation where you can fill your plate with healthy choices while helping yourself feel satisfied and full.

This approach helps you enjoy a variety of delicious and nutritious foods while still working towards your weight loss or health goals. It encourages you to fill your plate with wholesome ingredients rather than processed snacks or high-calorie options.

Key Features of the Zero Point Approach

1. **Focus on Nutrition:** Emphasizes whole, minimally processed foods that are high in nutrients.

2. **No Calorie Counting:** You don't have to count calories for Zero Point foods, allowing more freedom in your diet.

3. **Encourages Variety:** You can enjoy a wide range of foods, which helps keep meals interesting and enjoyable.

4. **Promotes Healthy Habits:** Helps you develop better eating habits by encouraging the consumption of fruits, vegetables, lean proteins, and whole grains.

While we'll get into the list of Zero Point foods later in this cookbook, it's important to understand that these foods typically include fresh fruits and vegetables, lean proteins like chicken and fish, and certain grains. The idea is to eat liberally from this list, allowing you to create delicious and satisfying meals without the stress of using up points.

The Zero Point Approach works by giving you a daily points budget based on your personal goals, activity level, and dietary needs. You'll track the points for the foods that are not Zero Point foods, which helps you maintain a balanced diet without feeling deprived. This system encourages you to make healthier choices, as you can consume as many Zero Point foods as you need to feel full.

For example, if you have a snack craving, you can grab an apple, some carrots, or a bowl of mixed greens without worrying about how many points you're using. The beauty of this approach lies in its flexibility. You can mix and match your meals and snacks, ensuring you never feel bored or restricted.

One of the biggest benefits of the Zero Point Approach is that it can make weight management feel less like a chore and more like a lifestyle. By focusing on foods that are good for you and satisfying, you can develop a healthier relationship with food. Plus, it can help reduce the likelihood of those pesky cravings that lead to overeating or unhealthy choices.

You might also notice that as you incorporate more Zero Point foods into your meals, you're naturally consuming fewer processed foods. This can lead to better overall health, increased energy levels, and potentially even improved mood over time.

CHAPTER 2
What Makes the Zero Point Approach Unique?

Unlike many other diets that have strict rules and limitations, the Zero Point Approach allows for much more flexibility in your food choices. Let's explore what sets this approach apart, making it a friendly option for those looking to improve their eating habits without feeling deprived2.

1. **Freedom of Choice**: Many traditional diets can feel restrictive, often requiring you to count every calorie or limit entire food groups. With the Zero Point Approach, you're encouraged to enjoy a wide variety of foods that are considered "Zero Point"—these are foods that don't add excess points to your daily tally. This means you can fill up on fruits, vegetables, and certain proteins without worrying about running out of points throughout the day.

2. **Focus on Nutritional Value**: While other diets may emphasize reducing calories at all costs, this approach encourages you to choose foods that are not only low in points but also packed with nutrients. This means you can savor whole, unprocessed foods that nourish your body, making it easier to maintain a healthy lifestyle.

3. **No Feeling of Deprivation**: Many diets can make you feel deprived, leading to cravings or even binge eating. The Zero Point Approach counters this by allowing a variety of foods that are satisfying and nutritious. When you're able to eat satisfying meals without the guilt of counting every point, you're less likely to feel the urge to snack on unhealthy options. This unique flexibility helps in creating a sustainable lifestyle change rather than just a temporary diet.

4. **Encouragement of Mindful Eating**: With the Zero Point Approach, there's a significant emphasis on mindful eating. This means taking the time to enjoy your meals, pay attention to your hunger cues, and appreciate the food you're consuming. Unlike diets that push you to focus solely on numbers, the Zero Point Approach invites you to engage with your food, making the process more enjoyable. This can lead to better digestion and a healthier relationship with food overall.

5. **Tailored for Individual Needs**: Every person is different, and the Zero Point Approach recognizes this by allowing you to tailor your eating habits to fit your lifestyle. Whether you're a busy parent, a student, or someone

with a hectic work schedule, you can adapt the Zero Point Approach to suit your needs. This means you can plan meals that work for your life, making it easier to stick with the program.

6. **Community and Support**: There are countless groups and forums where participants share their experiences, recipes, and tips. This community aspect can be incredibly motivating and encouraging, helping you stay on track and feel connected to others who are on a similar journey.

CHAPTER 3

Must-Have Tools for Easy Cooking

You might be excited to jump into the kitchen and whip up some delicious meals, but without the proper utensils and equipment, things can quickly become frustrating. Think about it: trying to cook without a sharp knife or a decent pan is like trying to write without a pen. It just doesn't work well.

Having the right tools not only makes cooking easier but also more enjoyable. Each tool has its own purpose, and when you have the right ones, you'll find that prep time is quicker, cooking is simpler, and cleaning up afterward is a breeze. Plus, with the right tools, you can experiment more, which is key to finding what you love in the ZeroPoint foods.

1. **Efficiency:** The right tools save you time. A good knife cuts faster and more accurately, while a reliable pot heats evenly, making your cooking process smoother.

2. **Safety:** Quality kitchen tools are designed with your safety in mind. A sharp knife is safer than a dull one because it requires less force to cut, reducing the risk of slips and accidents.

3. **Quality Results:** When you have the right tools, you can achieve better results. A good peeler, for example, can make prepping fruits and veggies a breeze, which means you can focus on flavor!

4. **Enjoyment:** Cooking should be fun! Using the right tools can take a lot of stress out of the process, allowing you to enjoy what you're doing.

Now that we've established why these tools are essential, here's my top picks for must-have kitchen tools that will make your cooking easier and more enjoyable.

TOOL	WHY YOU NEED IT	RECOMMENDATIONS
Chef's Knife	Essential for chopping, slicing, and dicing. A sharp knife is safer and faster.	Look for a 8-10 inch high-carbon stainless steel knife.
Cutting Board	Protects your countertops and provides a stable surface for cutting.	Choose a wooden or plastic board that's easy to clean.
Measuring Cups	Accurate measurements are key to consistent results.	A set of both dry and liquid measuring cups is ideal.
Mixing Bowls	Perfect for combining ingredients and easy to store.	Opt for stainless steel or glass options.
Spatula	Ideal for flipping, stirring, and serving.	A silicone spatula can withstand heat and is easy to clean.
Tongs	Great for flipping and serving food without making a mess.	Look for sturdy, heat-resistant tongs.
Peeler	Makes peeling fruits and veggies a breeze.	A Y-peeler is often easier to handle than a straight peeler.	
Can Opener	Essential for opening canned goods safely.	Choose a manual or electric one that's easy to use.
Colander	Perfect for draining pasta or rinsing fruits and veggies.	A sturdy stainless steel colander is versatile and durable.
Non-Stick Skillet	Excellent for cooking without sticking and easy cleanup.	A skillet with a ceramic non-stick coating is a healthy choice.

CHAPTER 4
How to Shop Smart for Zero Point Food

When you're shopping for Zero Point foods, you want to make sure you're not just grabbing whatever looks good. Smart shopping means making informed choices that align with your health goals while keeping your meal prep easy and enjoyable.

It's easy to get distracted by flashy packaging or convince yourself that a processed snack is a good idea just because it's labeled as "healthy." But with a little focus, you can navigate the aisles like a pro and come home with foods that actually benefit your body and your weight-loss journey.

1. **Plan Your Meals**: Before you even step into the grocery store, take some time to plan your meals for the week. This will help you stick to your shopping list and avoid impulse buys. Consider what recipes you want to try, and look for meals that include a variety of Zero Point foods. Write down your meals and create a shopping list based on what you need.

2. **Focus on Fresh Produce**: Fresh fruits and vegetables are your best friends when it comes to Zero Point foods. They're not only healthy but also versatile, making them great for snacks, sides, or main dishes. When shopping for produce:

    a)   *Choose Seasonal Items:* Seasonal fruits and veggies are often more affordable and taste better. Check your local farmers' market or grocery store for what's in season.

    b)   *Look for Bright Colors:* Aim for a colorful variety in your cart. The more colors you have, the more nutrients you're likely getting.

COLOR	SUGGESTED FOODS	BENEFITS
Green	Spinach, Broccoli	Rich in vitamins
Red	Tomatoes, Bell Peppers	High in antioxidants
Yellow/Orange	Carrots, Sweet Potatoes	Good for vision and skin
White	Cauliflower, Onions	Supports immune health
Purple	Eggplant, Beets	Contains anti-inflammatory properties

3. **Choose Lean Proteins**: Lean proteins are another essential component of the Zero Point food list. These include options like chicken breast, turkey, fish, and certain beans. When shopping for proteins:

a) *Check for Sales:* Look out for discounts or sales on lean meats. Stocking up when they're on sale can save you money.

b) *Consider Canned or Frozen Options:* Canned beans or frozen fish and chicken can be just as nutritious and often more affordable. Just be mindful of added sodium in canned products—look for low-sodium options when possible.

4. **Explore Whole Grains**: While many grains can be higher in points, whole grains like brown rice, quinoa, and oats can often be included as Zero Point foods in moderation. When adding grains to your shopping list:

a) *Buy in Bulk:* Purchasing grains in bulk can save you money and reduce packaging waste.

b) *Check for Whole Grains:* Look for labels that say "100% whole grain" to ensure you're getting the best nutritional value.

5. **Make the Most of Canned and Frozen Foods**: Canned and frozen foods can be lifesavers when it comes to convenience. They often have a longer shelf life and can be just as nutritious as fresh options. Here's what to keep in mind:

a) *Read Labels:* Choose options without added sugars or sauces. Look for canned vegetables that are low in sodium and frozen fruits without added sugars.

b) *Stock Up:* Having a variety of canned beans, tomatoes, and frozen veggies can make meal prep super easy.

Shopping for Zero Point foods doesn't have to be complicated. Stick to the basics, and don't feel pressured to try every new superfood out there. Focus on whole, unprocessed foods, and you'll be well on your way to a healthier lifestyle.

CHAPTER 5
Budget Friendly Shopping Tips

When it comes to sticking to a healthy eating plan without breaking the bank, following the Zero Point foods list is a fantastic way to keep your grocery budget in check. You might think that eating healthy and sticking to a specific list means you'll be spending a lot of money on fancy ingredients, but that doesn't have to be the case. In fact, there are plenty of budget-friendly shopping tips that make it easy to maintain a healthy lifestyle while staying wallet-friendly.

1. **Buy in Bulk**: Buying in bulk can be a great way to save money, especially for staple items that are Zero Point foods. Look for bulk bins in your grocery store for items like beans, lentils, and whole grains. These foods are not only budget-friendly but also nutritious and filling. If you have access to a warehouse store, consider purchasing larger quantities of Zero Point items to save even more.

2. **Seasonal Shopping**: Fruits and vegetables are essential for a balanced diet, and buying them in season can save you a lot of money. Seasonal produce is often less expensive and tastes better too. Check local farmer's markets for fresh, in-season produce at lower prices.

SEASON	FRUITS	VEGETABLES
Spring	Strawberries, Cherries	Asparagus, Spinach
Summer	Peaches, Watermelon	Zucchini, Cucumbers
Fall	Apples, Pears	Pumpkins, Sweet Potatoes
Winter	Oranges, Grapefruits	Kale, Carrots

3. **Use Coupons and Apps**: Don't forget to utilize coupons and grocery apps! Many stores offer digital coupons that can be easily accessed through their apps. Additionally, there are numerous coupon websites that can help you find deals on Zero Point foods. Combining coupons with sales can lead to significant savings, so keep an eye out for those promotions.

4. **Shop Generic Brands**: Generic or store-brand products are often cheaper than name-brand items and can be just as good in quality. When shopping for pantry staples like canned vegetables, frozen fruits, or spices, try opting for the store brand. You can save money without sacrificing quality, making it an easy switch for your budget-friendly shopping.

5. **Visit Local Markets:** Consider shopping at local markets or discount grocery stores. These places often have lower prices on fresh produce and pantry essentials compared to larger supermarket chains. Plus, you may find unique items that can add variety to your meals.

6. **Stock Up on Freezer-Friendly Items**: Freezing foods is a great way to preserve them and avoid waste. Items like fruits, vegetables, and even proteins can be frozen for future use. When you find great deals on these items, stock up. You can freeze portion sizes to help you create quick, easy meals later.

While it's essential to have a meal plan, being flexible can also save you money. If a specific ingredient is too expensive, look for alternatives that can achieve a similar flavor or nutritional profile. For example, if fresh herbs are pricey, consider using dried herbs instead.

Eating healthy with the Zero Point foods list doesn't have to be a burden on your wallet. By planning your meals, shopping smart, and being mindful of your purchases, you can enjoy nutritious foods without overspending. Remember, it's all about making choices that align with your budget while supporting your health journey.

CHAPTER 6
The Zero Point Foods List

The Zero Point can provide you with a sense of freedom in your diet. They're typically lower in calories but packed with nutrients, meaning you can fill your plate with satisfying meals without worrying too much about portion sizes. Plus, they're great if you're aiming to shed some pounds or maintain your weight while still enjoying delicious food.

When you know which foods are Zero Point, you can easily create meals that are not only healthy but also tasty. Let's be real: who wants to eat bland food? It's all about filling your plate with vibrant, flavorful ingredients that also happen to be good for you. This list will help you build a solid foundation for your meals, making it easier to stay on track with your health goals3.

1. **Fruits:** Fruits are not just delicious; they're packed with vitamins and minerals that your body loves. Think about adding berries to your breakfast oatmeal or snacking on an apple during the day. The natural sweetness helps satisfy your cravings without the added sugar.

2. **Vegetables:** Vegetables are your best friends on this journey. They add color, texture, and crunch to your meals. Try loading up on leafy greens like spinach or kale in your salads or smoothies. Roasted veggies are also a fantastic side dish—just add some herbs and spices for flavor!

3. **Proteins:** Protein is essential for keeping your body strong and energized. With options like chicken breast, fish, and tofu, you have plenty of ways to incorporate lean protein into your meals. A grilled chicken salad or a hearty vegetable stir-fry with tofu can be both satisfying and nutritious.

4. **Legumes:** Legumes are not only Zero Point foods but also a great source of fiber. They keep you feeling full longer and are perfect for soups, stews, or salads. Try adding black beans to your tacos or lentils to your soups for a hearty meal.

5. **Grains:** Whole grains are packed with nutrients and are a great way to fill your plate. Oats can be a wonderful breakfast option, while quinoa and brown rice work beautifully as a base for lunches or dinners. Don't forget to spice them up with your favorite seasonings!

6. **Dairy:** If you're a fan of dairy, you'll love that non-fat yogurt and cottage cheese are on the Zero Point list. They can be used in smoothies, parfaits, or even as a snack. Pair them with some fruit for added flavor and nutrition.

7. **Condiments:** Yes, you can enjoy your sauces too! Salsa, mustard, and vinegar can enhance the flavors of your dishes without adding points. A splash of vinegar can make a simple salad dressing, while salsa can brighten up any meal.

CATEGORY	ZERO POINT FOODS
Fruits	Apples, Bananas, Berries (all types), Oranges, Grapes, Pears, Pineapple, Peaches, Watermelon, Cherries, Plums, Kiwi, Mangoes, Strawberries
Vegetables	Spinach, Kale, Broccoli, Bell Peppers, Zucchini, Cucumbers, Carrots, Celery, Cauliflower, Green Beans, Asparagus, Mushrooms, Onions, Tomatoes, Sweet Potatoes, Brussels Sprouts
Lean Proteins	Chicken Breast (skinless), Turkey Breast, Fish (any kind, fresh, frozen, or canned), Shrimp, Shellfish, Tofu, Egg Whites, Tempeh
Legumes	Lentils, Chickpeas, Black Beans, Kidney Beans, Navy Beans, Pinto Beans
Whole Grains	Brown Rice, Quinoa, Oats (plain), Barley, Bulgur, Whole Wheat Pasta
Condiments & Spices	Mustard, Hot Sauce, Vinegar, Salsa, Garlic, Ginger, Fresh Herbs (like parsley, cilantro, basil), Lemon Juice, Lime Juice
Dairy Alternatives	Unsweetened Almond Milk, Unsweetened Soy Milk, Plain Greek Yogurt (non-fat)
Nuts and Seeds	(in moderation) – Almonds, Walnuts, Chia Seeds, Flaxseeds (be mindful of portion sizes)

Now that you've got a glimpse of the Zero Point food list, let's talk about how to use it in your daily life:

1. **Meal Prep:** Plan your meals around these foods. Fill your fridge with fruits and veggies from the list and always have some lean proteins on hand. This can help you whip up quick and healthy meals.

2. **Snacking:** Whenever you feel a snack attack coming on, reach for something from the Zero Point list. You can munch on raw veggies or some fruit without worrying about tracking points.

3. **Mindful Eating:** Since these foods are low in points, they allow you to be more mindful of portion sizes when indulging in higher-point foods. Pairing your favorite snacks with Zero Point options can help you enjoy them more without overdoing it.

Using the Zero Point food list can take your cooking and eating experience to the next level. Remember to check out the complete Zero Point foods list at the end of this cookbook for more options and ideas. You have an array of fruits, vegetables, proteins, grains, and condiments to choose from, and the best part is, you can mix and match freely!

CHAPTER 7

Breakfast Recipes

1. Zucchini & Tomato Egg Bake

Ingredients:

- 2 cups zucchini, diced
- 1 cup cherry tomatoes, halved
- 1 cup egg whites
- 1/2 tsp garlic powder
- 1/2 tsp salt (or to taste)
- 1 tbsp fresh basil, chopped

 Prep time: 10 min

 Cook time: 15 min

 Servings: 4

Directions:

1. Preheat your oven to 350°F (175°C).

2. In a mixing bowl, combine the zucchini, cherry tomatoes, garlic powder, and salt. Stir in the egg whites and basil.

3. Pour it into a greased baking dish, and bake for 15 minutes or until the egg whites are set.

Serving size: 1/4 of bake

Tips: Serve with a dollop of salsa for extra flavor and zero points!

Nutritional Values: Calories: 50; Carbs: 5g; Fat: 0g; Protein: 10g; Sugar: 3g; Sodium: 200mg; Fiber: 1g; Cholesterol: 0mg

2. Berry Blast Yogurt Parfait

Ingredients:

- 2 cups non-fat Greek yogurt
- 1 cup mixed berries
- 1 tbsp honey (optional)
- 1 tsp vanilla extract
- 1/4 cup granola (optional, for crunch)

 Prep time: 10 min

 Cook time: 0 min

 Servings: 2

Directions:

1. In a medium bowl, mix the Greek yogurt with vanilla extract and honey (if using).

2. In two serving glasses or bowls, layer half of the yogurt mixture at the bottom. Add half of the mixed berries on top.

3. Repeat the layering process with the remaining yogurt and berries. Top with granola for added crunch, if desired.

Serving size: 1 parfait

Tips: Swap out berries for any favorite fruit or seasonal options.

Nutritional Values: Calories: 150; Carbs: 20g; Fat: 0g; Protein: 15g; Sugar: 9g; Sodium: 60mg; Fiber: 3g; Cholesterol: 5mg

3. Egg White Breakfast Burrito

Ingredients:

- 1 cup egg whites
- 1/2 cup diced bell peppers
- 1/2 cup chopped spinach
- 1/4 cup diced onions
- 2 low-calorie whole wheat tortillas, warmed
- Salt and pepper to taste

Prep time: 10 min

Cook time: 15 min

Servings: 2

Directions:

1. In a non-stick skillet, sauté the diced onions and bell peppers over medium heat for 3-4 minutes. Add the spinach and cook for another minute until wilted.

2. Pour in the egg whites, season with salt and pepper, and scramble until fully cooked. Divide the egg white mixture evenly onto the tortillas, roll them up, and serve warm.

Serving size: 1 burrito

Tips: You can customize this recipe with your favorite veggies, such as mushrooms or zucchini.

Nutritional Values: Calories: 150; Carbs: 22g; Fat: 2g; Protein: 12g; Sugar: 1g; Sodium: 300mg; Fiber: 4g; Cholesterol: 0mg

4. Banana Oatmeal Muffins

Ingredients:

- 1 1/2 cups rolled oats
- 2 ripe bananas, mashed
- 1/2 cup unsweetened applesauce
- 1 tsp baking powder
- 1/2 tsp cinnamon
- 1 tsp vanilla extract

Prep time: 10 min

Cook time: 10 min

Servings: 6

Directions:

1. Preheat the oven to 350°F (175°C).

2. In a large bowl, mix rolled oats, bananas, applesauce, baking powder, cinnamon, and vanilla extract.

1. Spoon it evenly into the muffin tin, and bake for 15 minutes or until golden. Cool it down before removing from the tin.

Serving size: 1 muffin

Tips: Add a handful of walnuts or chocolate chips for extra flavor!

Nutritional Values: Calories: 110; Carbs: 22g; Fat: 1g; Protein: 3g; Sugar: 3g; Sodium: 5mg; Fiber: 3g; Cholesterol: 0mg

5. Peach & Ginger Yogurt Cup

Ingredients:

- 1 cup non-fat Greek yogurt
- 1 ripe peach, diced
- 1/2 tsp fresh ginger, grated
- 1 tsp cinnamon
- Almond slivers for topping (optional)

Prep time: 5 min

Cook time: 0 min

Servings: 1

Directions:

1. In a small bowl, combine the Greek yogurt with ginger and cinnamon until smooth. Gently fold in the peach, reserving a few pieces for topping.

2. Transfer the yogurt mixture into a serving bowl and top with reserved peach pieces and almond slivers, if desired.

Serving size: 1 cup

Tips: For a refreshing twist, chill the peaches in the fridge before adding them to your yogurt.

Nutritional Values: Calories: 120; Carbs: 15g; Fat: 0.5g; Protein: 10g; Sugar: 8g; Sodium: 50mg; Fiber: 3g; Cholesterol: 5mg

6. Egg White Omelet with Salsa

Ingredients:

- 1 cup egg whites
- 1/2 cup bell pepper, diced
- 1/2 cup spinach, chopped
- 1/4 tsp salt
- 1/4 tsp black pepper
- 1/4 cup salsa

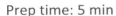

Prep time: 5 min

Cook time: 10 min

Servings: 1

Directions:

1. In a non-stick skillet, heat over medium heat. Add the bell pepper and cook for about 2-3 minutes until slightly softened.

2. Add the spinach and cook for 1 minute until wilted. Pour in the egg whites, salt, and pepper. Cook for 3-4 minutes, gently stirring until the eggs are set.

3. Slide the omelet onto a plate and top with salsa before serving.

Serving size: 1 omelet

Tips: For added flavor, sprinkle with fresh herbs or a dash of hot sauce.

Nutritional Values: Calories: 120; Carbs: 6g; Fat: 0g; Protein: 24g; Sugar: 2g; Sodium: 300mg; Fiber: 2g; Cholesterol: 0mg

7. Berry Chia Seed Smoothie Bowl

Ingredients:

- 1 cup frozen mixed berries
- 1 cup unsweetened almond milk
- 2 tbsp chia seeds
- 1 medium banana
- 1 tsp honey (optional)
- 1/2 cup sliced fresh fruit (for topping)

Prep time: 10 min

Cook time: 0 min

Servings: 2

Directions:

1. In a blender, combine the frozen mixed berries, almond milk, banana, and honey (if using). Blend until smooth.

2. Stir in the chia seeds and let sit for 5 minutes to thicken. Pour the smoothie into bowls and top with sliced fresh fruit.

Serving size: 1 bowl

Tips: Add a sprinkle of your favorite nuts or seeds on top for extra crunch!

Nutritional Values: Calories: 150; Carbs: 30g; Fat: 3g; Protein: 4g; Sugar: 8g; Sodium: 80mg; Fiber: 8g; Cholesterol: 0mg

8. Zucchini Bread Muffins

Ingredients:

- 2 cups shredded zucchini
- 1 cup whole wheat flour
- 1/2 cup unsweetened applesauce
- 1/2 cup zero-calorie sweetener (like stevia or monk fruit)
- 1 tsp baking powder
- 1 tsp cinnamon

Prep time: 15 min

Cook time: 20 min

Servings: 12

Directions:

1. Preheat the oven to 350°F (175°C) and line a muffin tin with paper liners.

2. In a large bowl, mix the zucchini, applesauce, and sweetener until combined.

3. Stir in the flour, baking powder, and cinnamon.

1. Pour the batter into the prepared muffin tin, and bake for 20 minutes or until a toothpick inserted comes out clean.

Serving size: 1 muffin

Tips: Keep leftovers in an airtight container for a quick grab-and-go snack!

Nutritional Values: Calories: 80; Carbs: 15g; Fat: 0.5g; Protein: 2g; Sugar: 1g; Sodium: 150mg; Fiber: 2g; Cholesterol: 0mg

9. Pumpkin Spice Oatmeal

Ingredients:

- 1 cup rolled oats
- 2 cups unsweetened almond milk
- 1 cup pumpkin puree
- 1 tsp pumpkin pie spice
- 1 tbsp maple syrup (optional)
- Pinch of salt

Prep time: 5 min

Cook time: 10 min

Servings: 2

Directions:

1. In a medium saucepan, let the almond milk boil. Stir in the rolled oats & salt.
2. Simmer for 5 minutes, stirring occasionally.
3. Add pumpkin puree and pumpkin pie spice, mixing well. Cook for 2-3 minutes until heated through.
4. If desired, add maple syrup for sweetness and stir. Serve warm.

Serving size: 1 bowl

Tips: For an extra flavor kick, top with a sprinkle of cinnamon or a few chopped nuts.

Nutritional Values: Calories: 150; Carbs: 28g; Fat: 2g; Protein: 5g; Sugar: 1g; Sodium: 15mg; Fiber: 4g; Cholesterol: 0mg

10. Breakfast Stuffed Spaghetti Squash

Ingredients:

- 1 small spaghetti squash (about 1.5 lbs.)
- 1 cup egg whites (or 4 large eggs)
- 1 cup diced bell peppers (any color)
- 1 cup diced tomatoes
- 1 tsp garlic powder
- Salt and pepper to taste
- Non-stick cooking spray

Prep time: 10 min

Cook time: 15 min

Servings: 2

Directions:

1. Preheat the oven to 400°F (200°C).
2. Cut the spaghetti squash in half lengthwise and scoop out the seeds.
3. Spray the inside of the squash with non-stick cooking spray and season with salt and pepper.
4. Place the squash halves cut-side down on a baking sheet and bake for 15 mins.
5. In a bowl, mix egg whites, bell peppers, tomatoes, garlic powder, salt, & pepper.
6. Flip the squash halves over, fill them with the egg mixture, and return to the oven for 10 minutes, or until the egg is set.

Serving size: 1 stuffed half of spaghetti squash

Tips: You can customize the filling with any of your favorite veggies.

Nutritional Values: Calories: 160; Carbs: 20g; Fat: 1g; Protein: 13g; Sugar: 3g; Sodium: 220mg; Fiber: 5g; Cholesterol: 0mg

11. Bell Pepper & Onion Frittata

 Prep time: 5 min   Cook time: 20 min   Servings: 4

Ingredients:

- 1 cup bell peppers, chopped
- 1 cup onion, chopped
- 1 cup egg whites
- 1 tsp garlic powder
- 1 tsp black pepper
- Salt to taste

Directions:

1. Preheat your oven to 375°F (190°C). In a large, oven-safe skillet, sauté the bell peppers and onions for 5 minutes over medium heat.

2. In a mixing bowl, whisk egg whites, garlic powder, black pepper, and salt.

3. Pour it over the sautéed vegetables in the skillet.

4. Cook on the stovetop for 5 minutes until the edges start to set, then transfer the skillet to your oven.

5. Bake for 15 minutes or until the frittata is set and slightly golden on top.

Serving size: 1 slice

Tips: Customize with your favorite herbs or spices for added flavor.

Nutritional Values: Calories: 70; Carbs: 4g; Fat: 0g; Protein: 15g; Sugar: 2g; Sodium: 150mg; Fiber: 1g; Cholesterol: 0mg

12. Breakfast Stuffed Spaghetti Squash

 Prep time: 5 min   Cook time: 0 min   Servings: 1

Ingredients:

- 1 cup non-fat Greek yogurt
- 1 medium apple, diced
- 1 tsp cinnamon
- Optional toppings:
- 1 tbsp honey
- 1 tbsp chopped walnuts
- 1 tbsp chia seeds

Directions:

1. In a bowl, scoop the Greek yogurt. Add the apple on top of the yogurt.

2. Sprinkle with cinnamon, stirring gently to combine.

3. If desired, drizzle with honey and sprinkle with walnuts and chia seeds for added texture. Serve.

Serving size: 1 bowl

Tips: For added flavor, try using different types of apples.

Nutritional Values: Calories: 200; Carbs: 30g; Fat: 4g; Protein: 18g; Sugar: 15g; Sodium: 80mg; Fiber: 5g; Cholesterol: 5mg

13.   Cheesy Spinach and Egg Bake

Prep time: 10 min   Cook time: 15 min   Servings: 4

Ingredients:

- 2 cups fresh spinach, chopped
- 1 cup egg whites (about 8 large egg whites)
- ¼ cup nutritional yeast
- 1 tsp garlic powder
- Salt and pepper to taste
- Cooking spray

Directions:

1. Preheat your oven to 350°F (175°C). In a large bowl, whisk egg whites, garlic powder, salt, and pepper.
2. Stir in the spinach and nutritional yeast until blended.
3. Pour the egg mixture into a greased 8x8 inch baking dish.
4. Bake for 15 minutes or until the egg is set and slightly golden on top.

Serving size: 1 square (1/4 of the bake)

Tips: Great for meal prep! Make it in advance and reheat for quick breakfasts throughout the week.

Nutritional Values: Calories: 60; Carbs: 2g; Fat: 0g; Protein: 12g; Sugar: 0g; Sodium: 200mg; Fiber: 1g; Cholesterol: 0mg

14.   Cauliflower Rice Breakfast Bowl

Prep time: 5 min   Cook time: 10min   Servings: 2

Ingredients:

- 2 cups cauliflower rice
- 1 cup egg whites
- 1/2 cup diced bell pepper
- 1/2 cup diced tomatoes
- Salt and pepper to taste
- Cooking spray

Directions:

1. Spray a non-stick skillet with a nonstick cooking spray over medium heat.
2. Add the diced bell pepper & sauté for 2-3 mins until slightly softened.
3. Stir in the cauliflower rice & cook for 5 minutes, stirring occasionally.
4. Push the cauliflower rice mixture to the side of the skillet and pour in the egg whites, cooking until scrambled and set.
5. Mix everything together and fold in the diced tomatoes. Season with salt and pepper, then serve.

Serving size: 1 bowl

Tips: Add your favorite herbs for extra flavor or incorporate leftover veggies for variety!

Nutritional Values: Calories: 80; Carbs: 6g; Fat: 3g; Protein: 10g; Sugar: 2g; Sodium: 250mg; Fiber: 3g; Cholesterol: 0mg

15.   Savory Cauliflower Porridge

Prep time: 10 min   Cook time: 15 min   Servings: 2

Ingredients:

- 2 cups cauliflower florets
- 1 cup low-sodium vegetable broth
- 1/2 cup unsweetened almond milk
- 1 tsp garlic powder
- 1 tsp onion powder
- Cooking spray

Directions:

1. In a large saucepan, spray the bottom with cooking spray and heat over medium.
2. Add cauliflower florets and cook for 2-3 minutes until slightly tender.
3. Pour in the broth and almond milk, then let it simmer.
4. Stir in garlic powder and onion powder.
5. Cook for an additional 10-12 minutes, stirring occasionally.
6. Remove and use an immersion blender to blend until smooth. Serve.

Serving size: 1 cup

Tips: You can add an egg on top for extra protein if desired.

Nutritional Values: Calories: 70; Carbs: 12g; Fat: 1g; Protein: 3g; Sugar: 2g; Sodium: 250mg; Fiber: 4g; Cholesterol: 0mg

16.   Breakfast Stuffed Spaghetti Squash

Prep time: 10 min   Cook time: 15 min   Servings: 2

Ingredients:

- 2 cups turnips, peeled and diced
- 1 cup spinach, chopped
- ½ cup mushrooms, sliced
- ¼ cup green onions, chopped
- 1 tsp garlic powder
- Cooking spray

Directions:

1. Spray a non-stick skillet with cooking spray & heat over medium-high heat.
2. Add the turnips & sauté for about 5 minutes until they start to soften.
3. Add mushrooms and cook for another 5 mins, stirring occasionally.
4. Stir in the spinach and garlic powder, then cook for an additional 3-4 minutes until the spinach is wilted.
5. Sprinkle with green onions & season with salt & pepper. Serve warm.

Serving size: 1 bowl

Tips: Customize with your favorite herbs or add sautéed vegetables for extra flavor.

Nutritional Values: Calories: 180; Carbs: 32g; Fat: 4g; Protein: 4g; Sugar: 1g; Sodium: 300mg; Fiber: 4g; Cholesterol: 0mg

17. Carrot Cake Overnight Oats

Prep time: 10 min   Cook time: 0 min   Servings: 1

Ingredients:

- 1/2 cup rolled oats
- 1 cup unsweetened almond milk
- 1/2 cup shredded carrots
- 1 tsp cinnamon
- 1 tbsp raisins (optional)
- 1 tsp vanilla extract

Directions:

1. In a mason jar or bowl, combine rolled oats and almond milk, stirring well. Add in the shredded carrots, cinnamon, raisins, and vanilla extract.
2. Cover and refrigerate overnight. In the morning, give it a good stir and enjoy cold or warm it up for a cozy breakfast!

Serving size: 1 jar

Tips: You can make several jars at once for a quick breakfast all week long.

Nutritional Values: Calories: 180; Carbs: 30g; Fat: 3g; Protein: 6g; Sugar: 5g; Sodium: 150mg; Fiber: 5g; Cholesterol: 0mg

18. Breakfast Stuffed Spaghetti Squash

Prep time: 10 min   Cook time: 15 min   Servings: 2

Ingredients:

- 2 cups fresh spinach, chopped
- 1 cup mushrooms, sliced
- 1 cup egg whites
- 1 tbsp onion powder
- 1 tsp black pepper
- Salt to taste

Directions:

1. In a non-stick skillet, sauté the mushrooms for 5 minutes over medium heat until they start to brown. Add the spinach and cook for about 2 minutes until wilted.
2. In a bowl, whisk egg whites, onion powder, black pepper, and salt. Pour it over the sautéed mushrooms and spinach.
3. Gently stir and cook for 3-5 mins until the eggs are fully cooked. Serve.

Serving size: 1 portion

Tips: For extra flavor, add a dash of hot sauce or sprinkle with fresh herbs.

Nutritional Values: Calories: 100; Carbs: 3g; Fat: 0g; Protein: 22g; Sugar: 1g; Sodium: 120mg; Fiber: 2g; Cholesterol: 0mg

19.   Zero Breakfast Energy Bites

Prep time: 10 min   Cook time: 12 min   Servings: 12 bites

Ingredients:

- 1 cup mashed ripe bananas (about 2 bananas)
- 1 cup blended chickpeas
- ½ cup powdered peanut butter
- ¼ cup unsweetened applesauce
- 1 tsp vanilla extract
- ½ cup chopped fresh fruit (such as berries or apple)

Directions:

1. Preheat your oven to 350°F (175°C). Line a baking sheet with parchment paper and lightly spray with cooking spray.
2. In a large bowl, mix mashed bananas, blended chickpeas, powdered peanut butter, applesauce, and vanilla extract.
3. Fold in the fresh fruit until evenly distributed.
4. Scoop out the mixture and form into small balls. Place them onto the prepared baking sheet.
5. Bake for 15 minutes or until lightly golden. Let cool before serving.

Serving size: 1 bite

Tips: Feel free to experiment with different fresh fruits for variety.

Nutritional Values: Calories: 55; Carbs: 12g; Fat: 1g; Protein: 2g; Sugar: 2g; Sodium: 35mg; Fiber: 2g; Cholesterol: 0mg

20.   Breakfast Stuffed Spaghetti Squash

Prep time: 10 min   Cook time: 15 min   Servings: 2

Ingredients:

- 3 cups grated cauliflower
- 2 large eggs
- ½ cup shredded carrots
- ¼ cup green onions, chopped
- ½ tsp garlic powder
- Salt and pepper to taste

1. In a large bowl, mix cauliflower, eggs, carrots, green onions, garlic powder, salt, and pepper. Heat a non-stick skillet over medium heat and lightly spray with cooking spray.
2. Scoop ¼ cup of the mixture into the skillet, flattening it into a hash brown shape. Cook for 4-5 minutes on each side until crispy. Repeat with the remaining mixture.

Serving size: 1 hash brown

Tips: Serve with a dollop of salsa or Greek yogurt for added flavor.

Nutritional Values: Calories: 70; Carbs: 6g; Fat: 3g; Protein: 5g; Sugar: 1g; Sodium: 50mg; Fiber: 2g; Cholesterol: 70mg

CHAPTER 8
Snacks and Appetizers

21. Watermelon Cucumber Gazpacho Shooters

Prep time: 10 min   Cook time: 0 min   Servings: 4

Ingredients:

- 2 cups watermelon, cubed
- 1 cup cucumber, peeled and diced
- 1 tbsp lime juice
- 1 tsp honey (optional)
- 1 tbsp fresh mint, chopped
- Salt and black pepper to taste

Direction.

1. In a blender, combine the watermelon, cucumber, lime juice, and honey (if using).
2. Blend until smooth. Season with salt and black pepper to taste.
3. Chill in the refrigerator for 15 minutes.
4. Serve in small glasses or shooters, garnished with chopped fresh mint.

Serving size: 1 shooter

Tips: For an extra refreshing twist, add a splash of coconut water before blending.

Nutritional Values: Calories: 40; Carbs: 10g; Fat: 0g; Protein: 1g; Sugar: 7g; Sodium: 5mg; Fiber: 1g; Cholesterol: 0mg

22. Tuna Celery Boats

Prep time: 15 min   Cook time: 0 min   Servings: 4

Ingredients:

- 1 can (5 oz) tuna in water, drained
- ½ cup plain non-fat Greek yogurt
- 1 tbsp Dijon mustard
- 1 tbsp lemon juice
- 4 stalks celery, cut into 3-inch pieces
- Salt and pepper to taste

Direction.

1. In a bowl, mix the drained tuna, Greek yogurt, Dijon mustard, lemon juice, salt, and pepper until well combined.
2. Spoon the tuna mixture into the celery sticks, filling them generously. Serve.

Serving size: 2 celery boats

Tips: Experiment with different spices, such as paprika or dill, for added flavor.

Nutritional Values: Calories: 60; Carbs: 3g; Fat: 1g; Protein: 11g; Sugar: 1g; Sodium: 150mg; Fiber: 1g; Cholesterol: 15mg

23.   Vegetable Crudité Platter

Prep time: 10 min   Cook time: 0 min   Servings: 4

Ingredients:

- 1 cup baby carrots
- 1 cup cucumber, sliced
- 1 cup bell pepper, sliced (any color)
- 1 cup cherry tomatoes
- 1 cup snap peas
- Your favorite zero-point dip (optional)

Direction.

1. Arrange all the vegetables artfully on a platter.
2. If desired, serve with a zero-point dip on the side.

Serving size: 1 cup of vegetables

Tips: Feel free to use any seasonal vegetables you have on hand. Pre-cut veggies can save time!

Nutritional Values: Calories: 50; Carbs: 12g; Fat: 0.5g; Protein: 2g; Sugar: 4g; Sodium: 50mg; Fiber: 4g; Cholesterol: 0mg

24.   Baked Kale Chips

Prep time: 10 min   Cook time: 15 min   Servings: 4

Ingredients:

- 1 bunch kale (about 8 oz)
- 1 tsp garlic powder
- 1 tsp paprika
- 1 tsp salt
- 1 tbsp nutritional yeast (optional)
- Cooking spray

Direction.

1. Preheat the oven to 350°F (175°C). Rinse the kale and dry thoroughly. Remove the thick stems and tear the leaves into bite-sized pieces.

2. In a large bowl, toss the kale with garlic powder, paprika, and salt until well-coated. Spread the kale evenly on a baking sheet. Lightly spray the kale with cooking spray to ensure even baking

3. Bake for 12-15 minutes, or until the edges are crispy but not burnt. Allow to cool before serving.

Serving size: 1 cup of kale chips

Tips: Keep an eye on the kale while baking to prevent burning. If you like it spicy, add a pinch of cayenne pepper!

Nutritional Values: Calories: 50; Carbs: 8g; Fat: 1g; Protein: 4g; Sugar: 0g; Sodium: 15mg; Fiber: 2g; Cholesterol: 0mg

25.   Cauliflower Buffalo Bites

Prep time: 10 min   Cook time: 15 min   Servings: 4

Ingredients:

- 1 lb. cauliflower florets
- 1/2 cup hot sauce (like Frank's RedHot)
- 1 tsp garlic powder
- 1/2 tsp paprika
- Salt to taste
- Cooking spray

Direction.

1. Preheat your oven to 425°F (220°C). Line a baking sheet with parchment paper and spray lightly with cooking spray.
2. In a large bowl, combine the cauliflower florets with hot sauce, garlic powder, paprika, and salt. Toss until evenly coated.
3. Spread the coated cauliflower on the baking sheet.
4. Bake for 15 minutes, or until the cauliflower is tender and slightly crispy.

Serving size: 1 cup

Tips: For extra flavor, try adding a sprinkle of nutritional yeast before serving.

Nutritional Values: Calories: 50; Carbs: 10g; Fat: 0g; Protein: 2g; Sugar: 0g; Sodium: 500mg; Fiber: 2g; Cholesterol: 0mg

26.   Tomato Basil Bruschetta

Prep time: 10 min   Cook time: 5 min   Servings: 4

Ingredients:

- 2 cups diced tomatoes
- 1/4 cup fresh basil, chopped
- 1 tbsp balsamic vinegar
- 1 tsp garlic, minced
- Salt and pepper to taste
- Cooking spray

Direction.

1. In a medium bowl, combine diced tomatoes, fresh basil, balsamic vinegar, and garlic. Season with salt and pepper.
2. Lightly spray it with cooking spray. Let the mixture sit for about 5 minutes. Serve on its own or on top of your favorite whole-grain or zero-point crackers.

Serving size: 1/2 cup

Tips: For an extra crunch, toast some whole-grain bread slices and top them with the tomato mixture.

Nutritional Values: Calories: 40; Carbs: 5g; Fat: 2g; Protein: 1g; Sugar: 3g; Sodium: 100mg; Fiber: 2g; Cholesterol: 0mg

27.   Cucumber Rounds with Zero-Point Hummus

Prep time: 5 min   Cook time: 0 min   Servings: 2

Ingredients:

- 1 large cucumber, sliced into ½-inch thick rounds
- ½ cup zero-point hummus
- 1 tsp paprika (optional)
- 1 tsp lemon juice (optional)
- Fresh herbs (like parsley or dill) for garnish (optional)
- Salt to taste

Direction.

1. Arrange the cucumber rounds on a plate. Top each round with a tbsp of zero-point hummus.

2. If desired, sprinkle paprika and lemon juice over the hummus. Garnish with fresh herbs and a pinch of salt.

Serving size: 4 cucumber rounds with hummus

Tips: For added flavor, try different zero-point hummus varieties, such as roasted red pepper or garlic.

Nutritional Values: Calories: 70; Carbs: 10g; Fat: 3g; Protein: 4g; Sugar: 2g; Sodium: 150mg; Fiber: 3g; Cholesterol: 0mg

28.   Spicy Roasted Chickpeas

Prep time: 10 min   Cook time: 0 min   Servings: 4

Ingredients:

- 1 can (15 oz) chickpeas, drained and rinsed
- 1 tsp smoked paprika
- ½ tsp cayenne pepper
- Salt to taste
- 1 tsp garlic powder
- Cooking spray

Direction.

1. Preheat the oven to 400°F (200°C). Pat the chickpeas dry with a paper towel to remove excess moisture.

2. Spray the chickpeas lightly with cooking spray and toss them with paprika, cayenne pepper, garlic powder, and salt until evenly coated.

3. Spread the chickpeas on a baking sheet. Roast for 15 minutes, shaking the pan halfway through, until crispy.

Serving size: ¼ cup roasted chickpeas

Tips: Store any leftovers in an airtight container for up to 3 days for a crunchy snack later.

Nutritional Values: Calories: 120; Carbs: 13g; Fat: 2g; Protein: 6g; Sugar: 1g; Sodium: 210mg; Fiber: 5g; Cholesterol: 0mg

29. Herbed Cauliflower Cakes

Prep time: 10 min   Cook time: 15 min   Servings: 4

Ingredients:

• 2 cups cauliflower florets, pulsed until they resemble rice or couscous

• 1/4 cup green onions, finely chopped

• 1/4 cup fresh parsley, chopped

• 1/4 cup egg whites (about 2 large egg whites)

• 1 tsp garlic powder

Cooking spray

Direction.

1. Preheat your non-stick skillet over medium heat and spray lightly with cooking spray.

2. In a bowl, mix cauliflower rise, green onions, parsley, egg whites, and garlic powder.

3. Form the mixture into small patties (about 2 inches wide) and place them in the skillet.

4. Cook for about 3-4 mins on each side or until golden brown. Serve warm

5. Remove from the skillet and serve warm.

Serving size: 1 cake

Tips: Pair these cakes with a zero-point yogurt dip for added flavor!

Nutritional Values: Calories: 50; Carbs: 8g; Fat: 0g; Protein: 4g; Sugar: 1g; Sodium: 50mg; Fiber: 2g; Cholesterol: 0mg

30. Jicama Sticks with Lime

Prep time: 5 min   Cook time: 0 min   Servings: 4

Ingredients:

• 2 cups jicama, peeled and cut into sticks

• 2 tbsp fresh lime juice

• 1/2 tsp chili powder (optional)

• 1/4 tsp salt

• Fresh cilantro for garnish (optional)

Direction.

1. In a bowl, toss the jicama sticks with lime juice, chili powder, and salt until evenly coated.

2. Arrange on a platter and garnish with fresh cilantro if desired. Serve.

Serving size: 1/2 cup

Tips: To add a twist, try using lemon juice instead of lime.

Nutritional Values: Calories: 35; Carbs: 9g; Fat: 0g; Protein: 1g; Sugar: 2g; Sodium: 50mg; Fiber: 4g; Cholesterol: 0mg

CHAPTER 9

Salad Recipes

31. Mixed Greens and Citrus Medley Salad

Prep time: 10 min   Cook time: 0 min   Servings: 2

Ingredients:

- 4 cups mixed salad greens
- 1 cup orange segments
- 1 cup grapefruit segments
- ¼ cup red onion, thinly sliced
- 1 tbsp apple cider vinegar
- 1 tsp Dijon mustard
- Salt and pepper to taste

Direction.

1. In a large bowl, combine the mixed greens, orange segments, grapefruit segments, and red onion.
2. In a small bowl, whisk the apple cider vinegar, Dijon mustard, salt, and pepper.
3. Drizzle the dressing over the salad and toss gently. Serve.

Serving size: 1 salad

Tips: For added flavor, sprinkle with fresh herbs like cilantro or mint.

Nutritional Values: Calories: 70; Carbs: 14g; Fat: 4g; Protein: 2g; Sugar: 7g; Sodium: 30mg; Fiber: 4g; Cholesterol: 0mg

32. Radish and Cucumber Salad

Prep time: 10 min   Cook time: 0 min   Servings: 2

Ingredients:

- 2 cups cucumbers, diced
- 1 cup radishes, thinly sliced
- ½ cup cherry tomatoes, halved
- 2 tbsp fresh dill or parsley, chopped
- 1 tbsp lemon juice
- Salt and pepper to taste

Direction.

1. In a medium bowl, combine the diced cucumbers, sliced radishes, cherry tomatoes, and fresh herbs.
2. Drizzle with lemon juice and season with salt and pepper. Toss well, then serve.

Serving size: 1 salad

Tips: This salad can be made in advance and stored in the fridge for up to a day.

Nutritional Values: Calories: 45; Carbs: 10g; Fat: 0g; Protein: 2g; Sugar: 3g; Sodium: 5mg; Fiber: 2g; Cholesterol: 0mg

33.   Cauliflower Rice and Herb Salad

Prep time: 10 min   Cook time: 15 min   Servings: 4

Ingredients:

- 4 cups cauliflower rice
- 1 cup diced cucumber
- 1 cup cherry tomatoes, halved
- 1/4 cup chopped fresh parsley
- 1/4 cup chopped fresh mint
- 2 tbsp lemon juice

Direction.

1. In a large bowl, combine the cauliflower rice, diced cucumber, cherry tomatoes, parsley, and mint.

2. Drizzle with lemon juice and toss until well mixed. Season with salt and pepper, then serve.

Serving size: 1 cup

Tips: For added flavor, consider tossing in a dash of your favorite spices like garlic powder or cumin.

Nutritional Values: Calories: 80; Carbs: 12g; Fat: 0.5g; Protein: 5g; Sugar: 3g; Sodium: 30mg; Fiber: 4g; Cholesterol: 0mg

34.   Pickled Onion and Avocado Salad

Prep time: 10 min   Cook time: 0 min   Servings: 4

Ingredients:

- 1 cup thinly sliced red onion
- 1 cup diced ripe avocado
- 2 tbsp white vinegar
- 1 cup mixed greens (e.g., arugula, spinach)
- 2 tbsp lime juice
- 1 tsp ground cumin
- Salt and pepper to taste

Direction.

1. In a small bowl, combine red onion and vinegar, allowing it to pickle for about 5 minutes.

2. In a separate bowl, combine avocado and mixed greens.

3. Add the pickled onions (drained), then gently toss to combine. Drizzle lime juice over the salad and sprinkle with ground cumin, salt, and pepper.

4. 3. Toss gently to combine, being careful not to mash the avocado. Serve.

Serving size: 1 cup

Tips: If you prefer a bit of heat, add a pinch of red pepper flakes to the dressing.

Nutritional Values: Calories: 120; Carbs: 9g; Fat: 15g; Protein: 4g; Sugar: 1g; Sodium: 60mg; Fiber: 7g; Cholesterol: 0mg

35.   Savory Cabbage and Apple Salad

Prep time: 10 min   Cook time: 0 min   Servings: 4

Ingredients:

- 4 cups green cabbage, shredded
- 1 large apple, diced
- 1/4 cup red onion, thinly sliced
- ¼ cup apple cider vinegar
- 1 tsp Dijon mustard
- Salt and pepper to taste

Direction.

1. In a large bowl, combine the shredded cabbage, diced apple, and sliced red onion.

2. In a small bowl, whisk together the apple cider vinegar, Dijon mustard, salt, and pepper.

3. Pour the dressing over the cabbage mixture and toss until well combined. Let it sit for a few minutes before serving.

Serving size: 1 cup

Tips: Add a sprinkle of nuts or seeds for extra crunch if desired.

Nutritional Values: Calories: 60; Carbs: 14g; Fat: 0.5g; Protein: 1g; Sugar: 2g; Sodium: 15mg; Fiber: 3g; Cholesterol: 0mg

36.   Bell Pepper and Chickpea Salad

Prep time: 15 min   Cook time: 0 min   Servings: 4

Ingredients:

- 2 cups bell peppers (any color), diced
- 1 can (15 oz) chickpeas, drained and rinsed
- 1/4 cup red onion, diced
- 2 tbsp lemon juice
- 1 tbsp fresh parsley, chopped
- Salt and pepper, to taste

Direction.

1. In a large bowl, combine the diced bell peppers, chickpeas, and diced red onion.

2. In a separate small bowl, mix together the lemon juice, parsley, salt, and pepper. Pour the dressing over the salad and toss gently to combine. Serve.

Serving size: 1 cup

Tips: For added flavor, consider including a pinch of cumin or your favorite spices.

Nutritional Values: Calories: 80; Carbs: 14g; Fat: 1g; Protein: 4g; Sugar: 2g; Sodium: 30mg; Fiber: 4g; Cholesterol: 0mg

37.   Radicchio and Endive Salad

Prep time: 10 min   Cook time: 0 min   Servings: 2

Ingredients:

- 2 cups radicchio, chopped
- 2 cups endive, chopped
- 1 cup cherry tomatoes, halved
- 1 cup cucumber, diced
- ¼ cup balsamic vinegar
- 1 tsp dried oregano
- Salt and pepper to taste

Direction.

1. In a large mixing bowl, mix radicchio, endive, cherry tomatoes, and cucumber.

2. In a separate small bowl, whisk together balsamic vinegar, dried oregano, salt, and pepper for the dressing.

3. Drizzle the dressing over the salad and toss gently to combine. Serve.

Serving size: 1 cup

Tips: Add a sprinkle of nutritional yeast for a cheesy flavor without adding points.

Nutritional Values: Calories: 50; Carbs: 10g; Fat: 0g; Protein: 2g; Sugar: 2g; Sodium: 10mg; Fiber: 3g; Cholesterol: 0mg

38.   Asparagus and Pea Salad

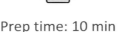

Prep time: 10 min   Cook time: 15 min   Servings: 2

Ingredients:

- 2 cups asparagus, cut into 1-inch pieces
- 1 cup frozen peas
- 1 cup cherry tomatoes, halved
- 2 tbsp lemon juice
- Salt and black pepper to taste

Direction.

1. In a medium pot, bring water to a boil. Add the asparagus and cook for 3 minutes until bright green and tender-crisp.

2. Add the peas and cook for 2 minutes. Drain and rinse under cold water.

3. In a large bowl, mix asparagus, peas, and cherry tomatoes. Drizzle with lemon juice, then season with salt and black pepper. Toss gently, and serve.

Serving size: 1 cup

Tips: Feel free to add fresh herbs like basil or mint for extra flavor!

Nutritional Values: Calories: 55; Carbs: 10g; Fat: 0g; Protein: 3g; Sugar: 3g; Sodium: 25mg; Fiber: 4g; Cholesterol: 0mg

39. Spicy Kale and Mango Salad

Prep time: 10 min   Cook time: 0 min   Servings: 2

Ingredients:

- 4 cups kale, chopped
- 1 ripe mango, peeled and diced
- 1 jalapeño, finely chopped
- 2 tbsp apple cider vinegar
- 1 tbsp honey (optional)
- Salt to taste

Direction.

1. In a large bowl, mix kale and salt. Massage the kale for 1-2 minutes until it starts to soften. Add the mango and jalapeño to the bowl.
2. In a small bowl, whisk together the apple cider vinegar and honey (if using). Drizzle the dressing over the salad and toss gently. Serve.

Serving size: 1 cup

Tips: Adjust the amount of jalapeño based on your spice tolerance, and consider adding nuts for crunch!

Nutritional Values: Calories: 85; Carbs: 16g; Fat: 1g; Protein: 3g; Sugar: 5g; Sodium: 30mg; Fiber: 3g; Cholesterol: 0mg

40. Shredded Vegetable Salad

Prep time: 10 min   Cook time: 0 min   Servings: 2

Ingredients:

- 2 cups green cabbage, shredded
- 1 cup carrots, grated
- 1 cup bell peppers, thinly sliced
- 1 cup cucumber, thinly sliced
- 2 tbsp apple cider vinegar
- 1 tsp Dijon mustard
- Salt and pepper to taste

Direction.

1. In a large bowl, combine the cabbage, carrots, bell peppers, and cucumber.
2. In a small bowl, whisk the apple cider vinegar and mustard.
3. Pour the dressing over the vegetables and season with salt and pepper. Toss gently, and serve.

Serving size: 1 cup

Tips: Add zero-point ingredients like chopped parsley or diced tomatoes for variety.

Nutritional Values: Calories: 45; Carbs: 9g; Fat: 0g; Protein: 2g; Sugar: 3g; Sodium: 30mg; Fiber: 3g; Cholesterol: 0mg

CHAPTER 10

Soups and Stews

41. Zucchini and Mint Soup

Prep time: 10 min   Cook time: 15 min   Servings: 4

Ingredients:

- 4 cups zucchini, chopped
- 1 cup onion, chopped
- 4 cups low-sodium vegetable broth
- 1 cup fresh mint leaves, packed
- Salt and pepper to taste

Direction.

1. In a large pot, add a splash of broth and sauté the onion over medium heat for 3-4 minutes until softened.

2. Add the zucchini and cook for 5 minutes, stirring occasionally. Pour in the broth and let it simmer. Cook for 10 minutes until the zucchini is tender.

3. Remove the pot and stir in the mint leaves. Blend the soup using an immersion blender until smooth. Season with salt and pepper, then serve.

Serving size: 1 cup

Tips: Garnish with a sprig of mint for an extra touch!

Nutritional Values: Calories: 50; Carbs: 10g; Fat: 0.5g; Protein: 2g; Sugar: 2g; Sodium: 300mg; Fiber: 2g; Cholesterol: 0mg

42. Cabbage and Beet Borscht

Prep time: 10 min   Cook time: 15 min   Servings: 4

Ingredients:

- 2 cups cabbage, shredded
- 1 cup beets, grated
- 1 cup onion, chopped
- 4 cups low-sodium vegetable broth
- 1 tbsp apple cider vinegar
- Salt and pepper to taste

Direction.

1. In a large pot, mix onion and shredded cabbage. Sauté over medium heat for 5 minutes until the onion is translucent.

2. Add the beets and vegetable broth. Let it boil, then adjust to a simmer for 10 minutes until the beets and cabbage are tender.

3. Stir in the apple cider vinegar and season with salt and pepper. Serve hot, with a sprinkle of fresh herbs if desired.

Serving size: 1 cup

Tips: For added flavor, top with a dollop of plain yogurt (optional).

Nutritional Values: Calories: 60; Carbs: 13g; Fat: 0g; Protein: 2g; Sugar: 4g; Sodium: 250mg; Fiber: 4g; Cholesterol: 0mg

43. Mushroom and Cauliflower Cream Soup

Prep time: 10 min   Cook time: 0 min   Servings: 2

Ingredients:

- 2 cups cauliflower florets
- 2 cups sliced mushrooms
- 1 medium onion, chopped
- 3 cups vegetable broth
- 1 tsp garlic powder
- Salt and pepper to taste

Direction.

1. In a large pot, sauté the onion in a splash of water for 3 minutes over medium heat. Add the mushrooms and cook for 5 minutes until they start to soften.

2. Stir in the cauliflower florets, broth, garlic powder, salt, and pepper. Let it boil. Adjust to a simmer for 15 minutes, or until the cauliflower is tender.

3. Puree the soup using your immersion blender until smooth. Serve warm.

Serving size: 1 cup

Tips: Garnish with fresh herbs or a sprinkle of nutritional yeast for added flavor.

Nutritional Values: Calories: 60; Carbs: 10g; Fat: 1g; Protein: 3g; Sugar: 2g; Sodium: 300mg; Fiber: 3g; Cholesterol: 0mg

44. One-Pot Minestrone

Prep time: 10 min   Cook time: 14 min   Servings: 4

Ingredients:

- 2 cups vegetable broth
- 2 cups diced tomatoes (canned, no added sugar)
- 1 cup diced carrots
- 1 cup diced celery
- 1 cup chopped spinach
- 1 tsp Italian seasoning
- Salt and pepper to taste

Direction.

1. In a large pot, let the broth simmer over medium heat.

2. Add the tomatoes, carrots, & celery. Cook for 5 mins, stirring occasionally.

3. Stir in the spinach and Italian seasoning. Season with salt and pepper to taste.

4. Simmer for an additional 10 minutes or until vegetables are tender.

5. Remove and let sit for a couple of minutes before serving.

Serving size: 1 cup

Tips: Add some freshly chopped herbs for extra flavor if time allows.

Nutritional Values: Calories: 50; Carbs: 10g; Fat: 0g; Protein: 2g; Sugar: 3g; Sodium: 250mg; Fiber: 3g; Cholesterol: 0mg

45. Eggplant and Tomato Stew

Prep time: 10 min   Cook time: 15 min   Servings: 4

Ingredients:

- 1 medium eggplant (about 1 lb.), diced
- 2 cups diced tomatoes (fresh or canned)
- 1 cup onion, chopped
- 1 cup vegetable broth (low-sodium)
- 1 tsp Italian seasoning
- Salt and pepper to taste

Direction.

1. In a large pot, add a splash of broth and sauté the onion for 5 minutes.
2. Add the eggplant and continue to sauté for another 5 minutes.
3. Stir in the tomatoes, Italian seasoning, and remaining broth.
4. Let it boil, then reduce heat and simmer for 15 minutes until the eggplant is tender.
5. Season with salt and pepper to taste before serving.

Serving size: 1 cup

Tips: Serve over a bed of steamed vegetables for a complete meal.

Nutritional Values: Calories: 70; Carbs: 15g; Fat: 0g; Protein: 2g; Sugar: 4g; Sodium: 150mg; Fiber: 4g; Cholesterol: 0mg

46. Cilantro Lime Chicken Soup

Prep time: 10 min   Cook time: 15 min   Servings: 4

Ingredients:

- 1 lb. boneless, skinless chicken breast, cubed
- 4 cups chicken broth
- 1 cup diced tomatoes (fresh or canned)
- 1 cup chopped cilantro
- 2 tbsp lime juice
- Salt and pepper to taste

Direction.

1. In a large pot, let the chicken broth simmer over medium heat. Add the cubed chicken breast and cook for about 10 minutes, or until the chicken is cooked through.
2. Stir in the diced tomatoes, chopped cilantro, and lime juice. Season with salt and pepper, and simmer for an additional 5 minutes. Serve hot.

Serving size: 1 cup

Tips: Top with avocado slices or a dollop of Greek yogurt for added creaminess.

Nutritional Values: Calories: 150; Carbs: 5g; Fat: 2g; Protein: 28g; Sugar: 1g; Sodium: 300mg; Fiber: 1g; Cholesterol: 70mg

47.   Vegetable and Mushroom Stir Stew

Prep time: 10 min   Cook time: 15 min   Servings: 4

Ingredients:

- 2 cups sliced mushrooms
- 1 cup diced bell peppers
- 1 cup broccoli florets
- 1 cup sliced snap peas
- 2 cups vegetable broth
- 1 tbsp low-sodium soy sauce (or tamari)

Direction.

1. In a large pot, heat a splash of vegetable broth over medium heat.
2. Add the mushrooms and sauté for 3 minutes until they start to soften.
3. Add the bell peppers, broccoli, & snap peas. Stir & cook for another 5 mins.
4. Pour in the broth and soy sauce, bringing the mixture to a simmer. Cook for 7 minutes, allowing the vegetables to remain vibrant and crisp.

Serving size: 1 cup

Tips: Feel free to add other zero-point vegetables such as spinach or kale for added nutrition.

Nutritional Values: Calories: 70; Carbs: 12g; Fat: 0g; Protein: 4g; Sugar: 2g; Sodium: 250mg; Fiber: 4g; Cholesterol: 0mg

48.   Cabbage and Turnip Stew

Prep time: 10 min   Cook time: 15 min   Servings: 4

Ingredients:

- 4 cups chopped cabbage
- 2 cups diced turnips
- 1 cup diced tomatoes (canned or fresh)
- 1 cup low-sodium vegetable broth
- 1 tsp garlic powder
- 1 tsp onion powder
- Salt and pepper to taste

Direction.

1. In a large pot, add a splash of vegetable broth & heat over medium-high heat.
2. Add the chopped cabbage and diced turnips, sautéing for about 5 minutes until they start to soften.
3. Stir in the diced tomatoes, vegetable broth, garlic powder, onion powder, salt, and pepper.
4. Let it boil, then reduce heat to low and simmer for another 10 minutes, stirring occasionally. Serve.

Serving size: 1 cup

Tips: Add a sprinkle of fresh herbs like parsley or dill for an extra burst of flavor!

Nutritional Values: Calories: 70; Carbs: 15g; Fat: 0g; Protein: 3g; Sugar: 3g; Sodium: 150mg; Fiber: 4g; Cholesterol: 0mG

49.   Moroccan Carrot and Chickpea Stew

Prep time: 10 min   Cook time: 15 min   Servings: 4

Ingredients:

- 4 cups diced carrots
- 1 cup diced onion
- 2 cups low-sodium vegetable broth
- 1 cup canned chickpeas (optional), rinsed and drained
- 2 tsp ground cumin

Direction.

1. In a large pot, add a splash of vegetable broth and sauté the onion over medium heat for about 2 minutes until translucent.
2. Add the carrots and stir well. Cook for an additional 2 minutes.
3. Pour in the broth and add the chickpeas (if using), cumin, and cinnamon.
4. Let it boil, then reduce the heat to low and let it simmer for 10-12 minutes, or until the carrots are tender. Serve hot.

Serving size: 1 cup

Tips: Feel free to adjust the spices according to your taste preferences.

Nutritional Values: Calories: 70; Carbs: 15g; Fat: 0g; Protein: 5g; Sugar: 4g; Sodium: 150mg; Fiber: 5g; Cholesterol: 0mg

50.   Light Dahl with Spinach

   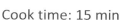

Prep time: 10 min   Cook time: 15 min   Servings: 4

Ingredients:

- 1 cup red lentils, rinsed
- 1 cup unsweetened almond milk
- 2 cups fresh spinach
- 1 tsp turmeric
- 1 tsp ginger (fresh or powdered)
- Salt to taste

Direction.

1. In a pot, combine the lentils, almond milk, turmeric, ginger, and salt. Add 2 cups of water and bring to a boil over medium heat.
2. Cover and simmer for 15 minutes, stirring occasionally, until the lentils are soft. Stir in the spinach until wilted. Serve warm.

Serving size: 1 cup

Tips: Serve with steamed cauliflower rice for a zero-point option.

Nutritional Values: Calories: 130; Carbs: 22g; Fat: 1.5g; Protein: 8g; Sugar: 1g; Sodium: 100mg; Fiber: 8g; Cholesterol: 0mg

51. Egg Drop Soup with Chicken

Prep time: 10 min   Cook time: 15 min   Servings: 4

Ingredients:

- 2 cups low-sodium chicken broth
- 1 cup cooked, shredded chicken breast
- 2 large eggs
- 1 cup spinach
- 1 tsp low-sodium soy sauce
- 1 tsp ginger (fresh or ground)

Direction.

1. In a medium pot, bring the chicken broth to a gentle simmer over medium heat. Add the shredded chicken, spinach, soy sauce, and ginger, stirring to combine.

2. In a small bowl, whisk the eggs until well beaten. Slowly pour the beaten eggs into the simmering broth while stirring gently to create egg ribbons.

3. Cook for an additional 2-3 minutes, then remove. Serve hot.

Serving size: 1 cup

Tips: Add chopped green onions or a sprinkle of sesame seeds for extra flavor.

Nutritional Values: Calories: 90; Carbs: 2g; Fat: 2g; Protein: 16g; Sugar: 0g; Sodium: 400mg; Fiber: 1g; Cholesterol: 150mg

CHAPTER 11

Grains, Pasta, and Rice Recipes

52. Black Bean Lentil Burgers

Prep time: 10 min   Cook time: 15 min   Servings: 4

Ingredients:

- 1 can (15 oz) black beans, drained and rinsed
- 1 cup cooked lentils
- 1/2 cup diced onion
- 1/2 cup diced bell pepper
- 1 tsp garlic powder
- 1 tsp cumin
- Non-stick cooking spray

Direction.

1. In a large bowl, mash the black beans with a fork until mostly smooth, leaving some chunks for texture.
2. Add the cooked lentils, onion, bell pepper, garlic powder, and cumin. Mix until well combined.
3. Form the mixture into 4 equal patties.
4. Spray a non-stick skillet with cooking spray and heat over medium heat.
5. Cook the patties for 4-5 minutes on each side or until golden brown and heated through.

Serving size: 1 burger

Tips: Serve with a side of mixed greens or your favorite zero-point dressing for a complete meal.

Nutritional Values: Calories: 120; Carbs: 22g; Fat: 0.5g; Protein: 8g; Sugar: 1g; Sodium: 300mg; Fiber: 7g; Cholesterol: 0mg

53. Cauliflower Gnocchi in Tomato Basil Sauce

Prep time: 5 min   Cook time: 15 min   Servings: 4

Ingredients:

- 1 bag (16 oz) frozen cauliflower gnocchi
- 1 cup canned crushed tomatoes
- 1/2 tsp dried basil
- 1/2 tsp garlic powder
- 1 tbsp nutritional yeast (optional)
- Salt and pepper to taste

Direction.

1. In a medium pot, bring water to a boil and add the frozen cauliflower gnocchi. Cook for 3-5 minutes until they float to the top. Drain and set aside.
2. In the same pot, add the crushed tomatoes, dried basil, garlic powder, and nutritional yeast. Stir to combine and let it simmer.
3. Add the gnocchi to the sauce and cook for an additional 5 minutes, stirring gently to coat the gnocchi in the sauce.

Serving size: 1 cup

Tips: Top with fresh basil or a sprinkle of red pepper flakes for extra flavor.

Nutritional Values: Calories: 140; Carbs: 26g; Fat: 2g; Protein: 4g; Sugar: 3g; Sodium: 350mg; Fiber: 4g; Cholesterol: 0mg

54.   Cauliflower Rice with Grilled Veggies

Prep time: 10 min   Cook time: 15 min   Servings: 4

Ingredients:

- 4 cups cauliflower rice
- 1 cup bell peppers, sliced
- 1 cup zucchini, sliced
- 1 cup cherry tomatoes
- 1 tsp garlic powder
- 1 tsp onion powder
- Non-stick cooking spray

Direction.

1. Preheat your grill or grill pan over medium-high heat.
2. Spray lightly with non-stick cooking spray.
3. Toss bell peppers, zucchini, and cherry tomatoes in garlic powder and onion powder.
4. Grill the vegetables for about 10 minutes, turning occasionally, until tender and slightly charred.
5. Meanwhile, in a separate skillet, warm the cauliflower rice over medium heat for about 5 minutes, stirring occasionally.
6. Serve grilled veggies over the cauliflower rice.

Serving size: 1 cup

Tips: Add fresh herbs like parsley / basil for extra flavor without additional calories.

Nutritional Values: Calories: 50; Carbs: 10g; Fat: 0g; Protein: 4g; Sugar: 2g; Sodium: 10mg; Fiber: 4g; Cholesterol: 0mg

55.   Cauliflower Rice and Beans Stuffed Peppers

Prep time: 10 min   Cook time: 15 min   Servings: 4

Ingredients:

- 4 large bell peppers (any color)
- 2 cups cauliflower rice (fresh or frozen)
- 1 can (15 oz) black beans, rinsed and drained
- 1 cup corn (fresh or frozen)
- 1 tsp cumin
- 1 tsp chili powder
- Salt and pepper to taste

Direction.

1. Preheat your oven to 375°F (190°C).
2. Slice the tops off the bell peppers and remove the seeds. Place them in a baking dish upright.
3. In a large bowl, combine cauliflower rice, black beans, corn, cumin, chili powder, salt, and pepper. Mix well.
4. Stuff each bell pepper with it, packing it tightly.
5. Cover the baking dish with foil and bake for 15 minutes, or until the peppers are tender. Serve warm!

Serving size: 1 stuffed pepper

Tips: Top with zero point salsa / a dollop of nonfat Greek yogurt for added flavor.

Nutritional Values: Calories: 130; Carbs: 28g; Fat: 0g; Protein: 6g; Sugar: 3g; Sodium: 200mg; Fiber: 9g; Cholesterol: 0mg

56. Lentil Salad with Roasted Vegetables

Prep time: 10 min   Cook time: 15 min   Servings: 4

Ingredients:

- 2 cups cooked lentils, drained and rinsed
- 1 cup cherry tomatoes
- 1 cup cucumbers, diced
- 1 cup bell peppers, diced
- 1 tbsp balsamic vinegar
- 1 tsp dried oregano

Direction.

1. Preheat your oven to 400°F (200°C).
2. On a baking sheet, toss cherry tomatoes and bell peppers with oregano and spray with non-stick cooking spray.
3. Roast the vegetables in the oven for about 15 minutes or until tender.
4. In a large bowl, combine cooked lentils, roasted vegetables, & diced cucumbers.
5. Drizzle with balsamic vinegar and toss gently to combine.

Serving size: 1 cup

Tips: Feel free to swap in any seasonal vegetables you have on hand!

Nutritional Values: Calories: 130; Carbs: 24g; Fat: 0g; Protein: 9g; Sugar: 4g; Sodium: 45mg; Fiber: 7g; Cholesterol: 0mg

57. Chickpea and Cauliflower Rice Buddha Bowl

Prep time: 10 min   Cook time: 15 min   Servings: 4

Ingredients:

- 1 cup canned chickpeas, drained and rinsed
- 2 cups cauliflower rice
- Splash of low-sodium vegetable broth
- 2 cups fresh spinach
- 1 cup diced cucumber
- 1 cup non-fat yogurt
- 2 tbsp lemon juice
- 1 tsp garlic powder
- Salt and pepper to taste

Direction.

1. In a large skillet, cook the cauliflower rice in a splash of broth over medium heat for about 5-7 minutes until tender.
2. Stir in the chickpeas and spinach, cooking for an additional 3-5 minutes until the spinach wilts.
3. In a small bowl, mix the yogurt, lemon juice, garlic powder, salt, and pepper to create the dressing.
4. Divide the cauliflower rice mixture into two bowls. Top with diced cucumber and drizzle the yogurt dressing over each bowl.

Serving size: 1 bowl

Tips: Add your favorite fresh herbs like parsley or cilantro for extra flavor!

Nutritional Values: Calories: 240; Carbs: 36g; Fat: 1g; Protein: 14g; Sugar: 5g; Sodium: 200mg; Fiber: 10g; Cholesterol: 0mg

58. Bulgur Wheat Tacos

Prep time: 10 min   Cook time: 15 min   Servings: 4

Ingredients:

- 1 cup bulgur wheat
- 2 cups vegetable broth
- 1 cup canned black beans, rinsed and drained
- 1 cup diced tomatoes
- 1 tsp cumin
- 1 tsp chili powder

Direction.

1. In a medium saucepan, let the broth boil. Add bulgur wheat, cover, and let it simmer for about 12 minutes, or until the liquid is absorbed.
2. In a large bowl, combine the cooked bulgur, black beans, diced tomatoes, cumin, and chili powder. Mix well.
3. Serve the bulgur mixture in lettuce wraps.

Serving size: 1 taco

Tips: Top with fresh avocado or cilantro for added flavor without extra points!

Nutritional Values: Calories: 150; Carbs: 28g; Fat: 1g; Protein: 6g; Sugar: 1g; Sodium: 200mg; Fiber: 7g; Cholesterol: 0mg

59. Spaghetti Squash Primavera

Prep time: 5 min   Cook time: 15 min   Servings: 4

Ingredients:

- 1 medium spaghetti squash (about 3 lbs.)
- 1 cup bell peppers, chopped
- 1 cup zucchini, sliced
- 1 cup cherry tomatoes, halved
- 1 cup broccoli florets
- 1 tsp garlic powder
- Non-stick cooking spray

Direction.

1. Preheat the oven to 400°F (200°C).
2. Cut the spaghetti squash in half lengthwise and scoop out the seeds.
3. Spray the inside of the squash with non-stick cooking spray and sprinkle with garlic powder.
4. Place the squash halves cut-side down on a baking sheet & roast for 20 mins.
5. Meanwhile, in a non-tick skillet, spray a bit of cooking spray and sauté the bell peppers, zucchini, cherry tomatoes, and broccoli over medium heat for 5 minutes until tender.
6. Once the squash is cooked, let it cool slightly, then use a fork to scrape the spaghetti-like strands into a bowl.
7. Mix the sautéed vegetables into the spaghetti squash and combine well.

Serving size: 1 cup

Tips: Sprinkle with fresh herbs / a squeeze of lemon for an extra burst of flavor!

Nutritional Values: Calories: 70; Carbs: 15g; Fat: 0g; Protein: 3g; Sugar: 3g; Sodium: 50mg; Fiber: 4g; Cholesterol: 0mg

60. Zucchini Noodles with Broccoli Rabe

 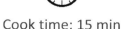

Prep time: 10 min   Cook time: 15 min   Servings: 2

Ingredients:

- 2 medium zucchinis, spiralized into noodles
- 2 cups broccoli rabe, chopped
- 1 tsp garlic, minced
- 1/2 tsp red pepper flakes (optional)
- Non-stick cooking spray
- Salt and pepper to taste

Direction.

1. Spray a non-stick skillet with cooking spray. Heat over medium heat.

2. Add garlic and red pepper flakes, and sauté for 1 minute until fragrant.

3. Add broccoli rabe and cook for 3-4 minutes until tender.

4. Add zucchini noodles, tossing everything together. Cook for an additional 4-5 minutes until the noodles are tender.

5. Season with salt and pepper before serving.

Serving size: 1 plate (approx. 1 cup)

Tips: For extra flavor, add a sprinkle of lemon juice or nutritional yeast before serving.

Nutritional Values: Calories: 70; Carbs: 12g; Fat: 1g; Protein: 4g; Sugar: 3g; Sodium: 150mg; Fiber: 4g; Cholesterol: 0mg

61. Cauliflower Rice with Grilled Chicken Bowl

Prep time: 10 min   Cook time: 15 min   Servings: 2

Ingredients:

- 2 cups cauliflower rice
- 1 lb. boneless, skinless chicken breast
- 1 cup bell peppers, sliced
- 1 cup zucchini, sliced
- 1 tsp garlic powder
- 1 tsp paprika
- Non-stick cooking spray

Direction.

1. Season the chicken breast with garlic powder, paprika, salt, and pepper.

2. Spray a non-stick skillet with cooking spray, then grill the chicken over medium-high heat for about 6-7 minutes on each side. Remove and let it rest.

3. In the same skillet, add the cauliflower rice and sauté for about 5 minutes until heated through.

4. Add the bell peppers and zucchini and cook for 3-4 mins until they are tender.

5. Slice the grilled chicken and serve it over the cauliflower rice and vegetable mixture.

Serving size: 1 bowl

Tips: Substitute the chicken for shrimp or tofu for a different protein option.

Nutritional Values: Calories: 270; Carbs: 16g; Fat: 3g; Protein: 52g; Sugar: 3g; Sodium: 300mg; Fiber: 5g; Cholesterol: 100mg

CHAPTER 12
Fish and Seafood

62. Chili Lime Grilled Shrimp Tacos

Prep time: 10 min　　Cook time: 10 min　　Servings: 4

Ingredients:

- 1 lb. shrimp, peeled and deveined
- 1 tbsp chili powder
- 1 tsp garlic powder
- 1 tbsp lime juice
- 1 head of romaine lettuce, leaves separated
- ½ cup diced tomatoes
- Non-stick cooking spray

Direction.

1. In a bowl, toss the shrimp with chili powder, garlic powder, lime juice, and a pinch of salt.

2. Spray a non-stick skillet with cooking spray & heat over medium-high heat.

3. Add the shrimp and cook for about 2-3 minutes on each side, or until they are pink and opaque.

4. To assemble, take a lettuce leaf, add a few shrimp, & top with diced tomatoes.

Serving size: 2 tacos

Tips: For extra flavor, add sliced avocados or a drizzle of hot sauce.

Nutritional Values: Calories: 140; Carbs: 5g; Fat: 1g; Protein: 27g; Sugar: 1g; Sodium: 150mg; Fiber: 1g; Cholesterol: 195mg

63. Baked Halibut with Tomato Basil Relish

Prep time: 10 min　　Cook time: 15 min　　Servings: 4

Ingredients:

- 1 lb. halibut fillets
- 1 cup cherry tomatoes, halved
- 1/2 cup fresh basil, chopped
- 1 tbsp balsamic vinegar
- 1 tsp garlic powder
- Non-stick cooking spray

Direction.

1. Preheat the oven to 400°F (200°C).

2. Spray a baking dish with non-stick cooking spray and place halibut fillets in the dish.

3. In a bowl, mix cherry tomatoes, basil, balsamic vinegar, and garlic powder. Spoon the mixture over the halibut fillets.

4. Bake for 15 minutes or until the fish flakes easily with a fork.

5. Serve the halibut topped with the tomato basil relish.

Serving size: 1 fillet with relish

Tips: Serve over a bed of greens for a complete meal.

Nutritional Values: Calories: 180; Carbs: 6g; Fat: 5g; Protein: 30g; Sugar: 3g; Sodium: 200mg; Fiber: 1g; Cholesterol: 70mg

64. Blackened Catfish with Cabbage Slaw

Prep time: 10 min   Cook time: 15 min   Servings: 2

Ingredients:

- 2 (6 oz) catfish fillets
- 1 tbsp paprika
- 1 tsp garlic powder
- 1 tsp onion powder
- 2 cups shredded cabbage
- 1 tbsp apple cider vinegar

Direction.

1. In a small bowl, mix paprika, garlic powder, onion powder, salt and pepper. Rub the spice mixture evenly over both sides of the catfish fillets.

2. Heat a non-stick skillet over medium-high heat and cook the catfish for 4-5 minutes on each side until blackened.

3. In a separate bowl, toss shredded cabbage with apple cider vinegar, salt, and pepper. Serve the blackened catfish atop a generous portion of the cabbage slaw.

Serving size: 1 catfish fillet with slaw

Tips: For extra flavor, add a squeeze of lime over the slaw before serving.

Nutritional Values: Calories: 220; Carbs: 9g; Fat: 7g; Protein: 37g; Sugar: 2g; Sodium: 350mg; Fiber: 3g; Cholesterol: 80mg

65. Garlic Lemon Prawns with Quinoa

Prep time: 10 min   Cook time: 15 min   Servings: 2

Ingredients:

- 1 lb. large prawns, peeled and deveined
- 3 cloves garlic, minced
- 1 lemon, juiced
- 1 cup cooked quinoa
- 1 tbsp fresh parsley, chopped
- Non-stick cooking spray

Direction.

1. Spray a non-stick skillet with cooking spray and heat over medium-high heat. Sauté for 1 minute until fragrant.

2. Add the prawns and cook for 2-3 minutes until they turn pink. Squeeze lemon juice over the prawns, season with salt and pepper, and stir to combine.

3. Serve the garlic lemon prawns over cooked quinoa, garnished with fresh parsley.

Serving size: ½ lb. prawns with quinoa

Tips: Substitute quinoa with cauliflower rice for a lower-carb option.

Nutritional Values: Calories: 300; Carbs: 28g; Fat: 10g; Protein: 24g; Sugar: 1g; Sodium: 450mg; Fiber: 3g; Cholesterol: 190mg

66. Fish Tandoori Skewers

Prep time: 10 min   **Cook time: 15 min**   **Servings: 4**

Ingredients:

- 1 lb. firm white fish (like cod or tilapia), cut into chunks
- 2 tbsp tandoori spice mix
- 1 tbsp lemon juice
- 1 red bell pepper, cut into chunks
- 1 zucchini, sliced
- Salt and pepper to taste

Direction.

1. In a bowl, combine the fish chunks with tandoori spice mix and lemon juice. Thread the fish, bell pepper, and zucchini onto skewers, alternating ingredients.
2. Preheat the grill or grill pan over medium-high heat.
3. Season the skewers with salt and pepper, then grill for about 5-7 minutes on each side, or until the fish is cooked. Serve.

Serving size: 1 skewer

Tips: Soak wooden skewers in water for 30 minutes before grilling to prevent burning.

Nutritional Values: Calories: 150; Carbs: 5g; Fat: 2g; Protein: 28g; Sugar: 2g; Sodium: 150mg; Fiber: 2g; Cholesterol: 70mg

67. Sardine and Avocado Salad

Prep time: 10 min   **Cook time: 0 min**   **Servings: 2**

Ingredients:

- 1 can (about 4 oz) sardines in water, drained
- ½ cup avocado, diced
- 1 cup cherry tomatoes, halved
- 2 cups mixed greens
- 1 tbsp lemon juice
- Salt and pepper to taste

Direction.

1. In a large bowl, combine the sardines, avocado, and cherry tomatoes. Add the mixed greens and drizzle with lemon juice.
2. Gently toss to combine, adding salt and pepper. Serve immediately.

Serving size: 1 bowl

Tips: For added crunch, toss in some chopped cucumber.

Nutritional Values: Calories: 200; Carbs: 10g; Fat: 9g; Protein: 22g; Sugar: 1g; Sodium: 300mg; Fiber: 4g; Cholesterol: 60mg

68. Seafood Chowder with Cauliflower Base

Prep time: 15 min   Cook time: 10 min   Servings: 4

Ingredients:

- 4 cups cauliflower florets
- 2 cups seafood mix (shrimp, scallops, and calamari)
- 3 cups low-sodium vegetable broth
- 1 cup unsweetened almond milk
- 1 tsp garlic powder
- Salt and pepper to taste

Direction.

1. In a large pot, steam the cauliflower florets for 5-7 minutes until tender. Add the broth and almond milk, then blend until smooth using an immersion blender.

2. Stir in the seafood mix and garlic powder, then let the chowder simmer for 5 minutes, until the seafood is cooked through. Season with salt and pepper before serving.

Serving size: 1 bowl

Tips: Feel free to substitute any seafood you prefer or have on hand.

Nutritional Values: Calories: 150; Carbs: 10g; Fat: 4g; Protein: 18g; Sugar: 2g; Sodium: 300mg; Fiber: 3g; Cholesterol: 50mg

69. Baked Salmon with Dill Yogurt Sauce

Prep time: 10 min   Cook time: 15 min   Servings: 2

Ingredients:

- 1 lb. salmon fillet
- 1 cup non-fat Greek yogurt
- 2 tbsp fresh dill, chopped
- 1 tbsp lemon juice
- Salt and pepper to taste
- 1 tsp garlic powder

Direction.

1. Preheat the oven to 400°F (200°C). Place the salmon fillet on a lined baking sheet. Season with salt, pepper, and garlic powder.

2. Bake the salmon for about 12-15 minutes, or until it flakes easily.

3. Meanwhile, mix the Greek yogurt, dill, lemon juice, and a pinch of salt in a small bowl to create the sauce.

4. Serve the baked salmon topped with the dill yogurt sauce.

Serving size: 1/4 of the salmon fillet with sauce

Tips: You can make the sauce ahead of time and store it in the fridge for up to 3 days.

Nutritional Values: Calories: 210; Carbs: 3g; Fat: 8g; Protein: 32g; Sugar: 1g; Sodium: 120mg; Fiber: 0g; Cholesterol: 80mg

70. Sautéed Scallops with Asparagus

Prep time: 10 min   Cook time: 10 min   Servings: 2

Ingredients:

- 1 lb. scallops, cleaned
- 2 cups asparagus, trimmed and cut into 1-inch pieces
- Non-stick cooking spray
- 2 cloves garlic, minced
- 1 tsp lemon juice
- Salt and pepper to taste

Direction.

1. Preheat a non-stick skillet over medium-high heat and lightly spray with non-stick cooking spray.

2. Add the asparagus and sauté for about 3 minutes until bright green. Remove and set aside.

3. In the same skillet, add the scallops, garlic powder, lemon juice, salt, and pepper. Cook for about 3-4 minutes or until the scallops are golden brown, flipping halfway through.

4. Return the asparagus to the skillet, and cook for an additional 1-2 minutes to heat through. Serve.

Serving size: 1 plate

Tips: Ensure scallops are dry before cooking for a better sear.

Nutritional Values: Calories: 180; Carbs: 6g; Fat: 2g; Protein: 32g; Sugar: 2g; Sodium: 250mg; Fiber: 2g; Cholesterol: 40mg

71. Coconut Curry Lobster

 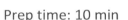

Prep time: 10 min   Cook time: 15 min   Servings: 2

Ingredients:

- 1 lb. lobster meat, cooked and chopped
- 1 cup light coconut milk (or a blend of light coconut milk and vegetable broth)
- 2 tbsp red curry paste
- 1 cup bell peppers, sliced
- 1 cup spinach
- Salt to taste

Direction.

1. In a large skillet, heat light coconut milk over medium heat. Add red curry paste, stirring until well combined.

2. Add bell peppers and cook for 5 minutes until slightly tender. Stir in lobster meat and cook for an additional 5 minutes.

3. Add fresh spinach and cook until wilted. Season with salt and serve warm.

Serving size: 1 bowl (about 1.5 cups of lobster curry)

Tips: Serve over cauliflower rice for a fulfilling meal without added points.

Nutritional Values: Calories: 250; Carbs: 10g; Fat: 9g; Protein: 36g; Sugar: 2g; Sodium: 150mg; Fiber: 3g; Cholesterol: 70mg

72. Grilled Swordfish with Mango Salsa

Prep time: 10 min   Cook time: 10 min   Servings: 2

Ingredients:

- 2 swordfish steaks (about 1 lb.)
- 1 cup diced fresh mango
- 1/2 cup diced red onion
- 1/4 cup chopped fresh cilantro
- 1 lime (juiced)
- Salt and pepper to taste

Direction.

1. Preheat the grill to medium-high heat.

2. In a bowl, combine the mango, red onion, cilantro, lime juice, and season with salt and pepper to create the mango salsa. Set aside.

3. Season the swordfish steaks with salt and pepper. Grill the swordfish for about 4-5 minutes on each side, or until cooked.

4. Serve the grilled swordfish topped with the fresh mango salsa.

Serving size: 1 steak with salsa

Tips: For added flavor, marinate the swordfish in lime juice and spices for 15 minutes before grilling.

Nutritional Values: Calories: 230; Carbs: 14g; Fat: 10g; Protein: 28g; Sugar: 8g; Sodium: 150mg; Fiber: 2g; Cholesterol: 70mg

73. Teriyaki Glazed Mahi Mahi

Prep time: 10 min   Cook time: 15 min   Servings: 2

Ingredients:

- 1 lb. Mahi Mahi fillets
- 1/4 cup reduced-sodium teriyaki sauce
- 2 cups broccoli florets
- Non-stick cooking spray
- 1 tsp garlic powder
- 1 tsp ground ginger

Direction.

1. Preheat a non-stick skillet over medium heat. Lightly spray with non-stick cooking spray.

2. Season the Mahi Mahi fillets with garlic powder and ground ginger.

3. Place the seasoned fillets in the skillet and cook for about 5-6 minutes on each side, or until the fish flakes easily.

4. Meanwhile, steam the broccoli florets in a microwave-safe dish with a small amount of water for 3-4 minutes, until tender but still bright green.

5. During the last minute of cooking for the Mahi Mahi, drizzle the teriyaki sauce over the fillets and let it caramelize slightly.

6. Serve the glazed Mahi Mahi with steamed broccoli on the side.

Serving size: 1 fillet with broccoli

Tips: For a quick side dish, use pre-steamed broccoli from the grocery store.

Nutritional Values: Calories: 230; Carbs: 10g; Fat: 4g; Protein: 40g; Sugar: 4g; Sodium: 350mg; Fiber: 4g; Cholesterol: 70mg

CHAPTER 13

Poultry Recipes

74. Savory Chicken and Mushroom Skillet

Prep time: 10 min   Cook time: 15 min   Servings: 4

Ingredients:

- 1 lb. boneless, skinless chicken breast, diced
- 2 cups sliced mushrooms
- 1 cup low-sodium chicken broth
- 1 cup chopped spinach
- 1 tsp garlic powder
- Salt and pepper to taste

Direction.

1. In a large skillet, heat a non-stick pan over medium heat. Add the chicken breast and season with salt, pepper, and garlic powder. Sauté for 5 minutes until the chicken is browned.

2. Add the mushrooms to the skillet and continue to cook for another 5 minutes, stirring occasionally.

3. Pour in the broth and add the spinach. Let it simmer and cook for an additional 5 minutes until the spinach is wilted. Serve hot.

Serving size: 1 cup

Tips: Pair with a side salad for a complete meal!

Nutritional Values: Calories: 150; Carbs: 4g; Fat: 2g; Protein: 28g; Sugar: 1g; Sodium: 300mg; Fiber: 1g; Cholesterol: 70mg

75. Buffalo Chicken Lettuce Wraps

Prep time: 10 min   Cook time: 15 min   Servings: 4

Ingredients:

- 1 lb. shredded cooked chicken
- 1/2 cup low-calorie buffalo sauce
- 1 cup diced celery
- 1 cup diced carrots
- 1 head of romaine lettuce (for wraps)
- Salt and pepper to taste

Direction.

1. In a medium mixing bowl, combine the shredded chicken and buffalo sauce, stirring until the chicken is well coated.

2. Heat a non-stick skillet over medium heat and add the buffalo chicken mixture. Cook for 5-7 minutes, stirring occasionally.

3. Meanwhile, prepare the lettuce leaves by washing & separating them. Remove the skillet, & stir in the celery and carrots. Season with salt & pepper.

4. Spoon the buffalo chicken mixture into the lettuce leaves & serve immediately.

Serving size: 2 wraps

Tips: Add a dollop of Greek yogurt for an extra creamy texture!

Nutritional Values: Calories: 180; Carbs: 6g; Fat: 4g; Protein: 30g; Sugar: 1g; Sodium: 350mg; Fiber: 2g; Cholesterol: 80mg

76.   Mediterranean Chicken Skewers

Prep time: 10 min   Cook time: 15 min   Servings: 4

Ingredients:

- 1 lb. boneless, skinless chicken breast, cubed
- 1 cup cherry tomatoes
- 1 cup bell peppers, cubed
- 1 cup zucchini, sliced
- Non-stick cooking spray
- 1 tbsp dried oregano

Direction.

1. Preheat your grill or grill pan over medium-high heat.

2. In a large bowl, combine the chicken, cherry tomatoes, zucchini, bell peppers, oregano, and garlic powder.

3. Thread the chicken & vegetables onto skewers, alternating between chicken & veggies.

4. Lightly spray the grill with non-stick cooking spray. Grill the skewers for about 10-12 mins, turning occasionally, until the chicken is cooked through.

5. Remove from grill and let cool for a couple of minutes before serving.

Serving size: 1 skewer

Tips: Serve with a squeeze of fresh lemon juice for added flavor!

Nutritional Values: Calories: 180; Carbs: 8g; Fat: 6g; Protein: 25g; Sugar: 3g; Sodium: 70mg; Fiber: 2g; Cholesterol: 70mg

77.   Herbed Chicken Quinoa Bowl

Prep time: 10 min   Cook time: 15 min   Servings: 2

Ingredients:

- 1 lb. boneless, skinless chicken breast, diced
- 1/2 cup quinoa, rinsed
- 2 cups low-sodium chicken broth
- 1 cup cherry tomatoes, halved
- 1 cup fresh spinach
- 1 tsp garlic powder
- 1 tsp dried Italian herbs (basil, oregano, thyme)

Direction.

1. 1. In a medium saucepan, combine quinoa and chicken broth. Let it boil, cover, and simmer for 15 minutes until quinoa is fluffy.

2. Meanwhile, spray a non-stick skillet with cooking spray and heat over medium-high heat. Add diced chicken and season with garlic powder, Italian herbs, and salt to taste.

3. Cook chicken for about 7-10 mins until fully cooked and no longer pink.

4. Stir in cherry tomatoes & fresh spinach, cooking for 2 mins until spinach wilts.

5. Serve the herbed chicken mixture over the quinoa.

Serving size: 1 bowl (1/2 cup)

Tips: Feel free to add your favorite veggies on the side for extra nutrition.

Nutritional Values: Calories: 340; Carbs: 34g; Fat: 4g; Protein: 45g; Sugar: 2g; Sodium: 350mg; Fiber: 5g; Cholesterol: 70mg

78. Miso Glazed Chicken Thighs

Prep time: 10 min   Cook time: 15 min   Servings: 4

Ingredients:

- 1.5 lbs. boneless, skinless chicken thighs
- 1/4 cup miso paste (preferably a low-sodium variety)
- 2 tbsp sugar-free sweetener (e.g., erythritol, Stevia)
- 2 tbsp rice vinegar
- 1 tbsp low-sodium soy sauce
- Non-stick cooking spray

Direction.

1. In a bowl, mix the miso paste, sugar-free sweetener, rice vinegar, and soy sauce to create the glaze.
2. Preheat a non-stick skillet over medium heat and spray with cooking spray.
3. Add the chicken thighs and cook for about 6-7 minutes on each side.
4. Brush the miso glaze onto the chicken during the last 2 minutes of cooking, ensuring it's well-coated.
5. Remove and let rest for a couple of minutes before slicing.

Serving size: 1 thigh

Tips: Serve with a side of steamed vegetables or a fresh salad to round out your meal.

Nutritional Values: Calories: 180; Carbs: 3g; Fat: 7g; Protein: 24g; Sugar: 1g; Sodium: 400mg; Fiber: 0g; Cholesterol: 90mg

79. Glazed Garlic Chicken Drumsticks

Prep time: 5 min   Cook time: 20 min   Servings: 4

Ingredients:

- 2 lbs. chicken drumsticks
- 1/4 cup coconut aminos or low-sodium soy sauce (in moderation)
- 1 tbsp minced garlic
- 1 tbsp monk fruit sweetener or stevia
- 1 tsp ground ginger
- Non-stick cooking spray

Direction.

1. Preheat your oven to 400°F (200°C).
2. In a bowl, mix the coconut aminos, garlic, monk fruit sweetener, and ground ginger to create the glaze.
3. Spray a baking dish with non-stick cooking spray and place the chicken drumsticks in it.
4. Pour the glaze over the drumsticks, ensuring they are well coated.
5. Bake for 25 mins or until the chicken is cooked and slightly caramelized.

Serving size: 1 drumstick

Tips: You can also grill the drumsticks for a smoky flavor.

Nutritional Values: Calories: 180; Carbs: 4g; Fat: 6g; Protein: 28g; Sugar: 0g; Sodium: 290mg; Fiber: 0g; Cholesterol: 80mg

80. Turkey Cabbage Roll Casserole

Prep time: 10 min   Cook time: 25 min   Servings: 6

Ingredients:

- 1 lb. lean ground turkey
- 4 cups chopped green cabbage
- 1 cup diced tomatoes (canned)
- 1 cup onion, chopped
- 2 tsp garlic powder
- 1 tbsp Italian seasoning

Direction.

1. Preheat your oven to 375°F (190°C). In a large skillet, cook the ground turkey and onions over medium heat until the turkey is browned. Drain any excess fat.

2. Stir in the chopped cabbage, diced tomatoes, garlic powder, and Italian seasoning. Cook for 5 more minutes until the cabbage is slightly wilted.

3. Transfer the mixture to a baking dish and bake for 15 minutes until everything is heated through. Serve.

Serving size: 1 cup

Tips: Add a sprinkle of low-fat cheese on top during the last 5 minutes of baking for extra flavor.

Nutritional Values: Calories: 150; Carbs: 10g; Fat: 6g; Protein: 20g; Sugar: 3g; Sodium: 80mg; Fiber: 3g; Cholesterol: 60mg

81. Turkey and Quinoa Stuffed Zucchini

Prep time: 10 min   Cook time: 15 min   Servings: 4

Ingredients:

- 2 medium zucchinis, halved and scooped out
- 1 lb. ground turkey
- 1 cup cooked quinoa
- 1 cup diced tomatoes
- 1 tsp garlic powder
- Salt and pepper to taste

Direction.

1. Preheat your oven to 375°F (190°C). In a skillet over medium heat, cook the ground turkey for 5-7 minutes until browned. Drain any excess fat.

2. Stir in the cooked quinoa, diced tomatoes, garlic powder, salt, and pepper. Cook for another 2-3 minutes until heated through.

3. Spoon the turkey and quinoa mixture into the zucchini halves and place them in a baking dish. Bake for 10-12 minutes until the zucchini is tender.

Serving size: 1 stuffed zucchini half

Tips: Experiment with different spices or add chopped herbs for extra flavor.

Nutritional Values: Calories: 180; Carbs: 14g; Fat: 6g; Protein: 22g; Sugar: 3g; Sodium: 150mg; Fiber: 3g; Cholesterol: 70mg

82.   Garlic and Rosemary Roast Turkey Breast

Prep time: 10 min   Cook time: 15 min   Servings: 4

Ingredients:

- 1 lb. turkey breast, skinless
- 1 tbsp fresh rosemary, chopped
- 3 cloves garlic, minced
- 1 tsp salt
- 1 tsp black pepper
- Non-stick cooking spray

Direction.

1. Preheat your oven to 375°F (190°C).
2. Lightly spray a baking dish with non-stick cooking spray.
3. In a small bowl, mix the rosemary, garlic, salt, and pepper.
4. Rub the garlic and rosemary mixture all over the turkey breast.
5. Place the turkey breast in the baking dish and roast in the oven for 15 mins.
6. Let it rest for a few minutes before slicing.

Serving size: 4 oz of turkey breast

Tips: Pair with steamed veggies or a salad for a complete meal.

Nutritional Values: Calories: 140; Carbs: 0g; Fat: 2g; Protein: 30g; Sugar: 0g; Sodium: 300mg; Fiber: 0g; Cholesterol: 90mg

83.   Turkey Meatballs with Marinara

Prep time: 10 min   Cook time: 15 min   Servings: 4

Ingredients:

- 1 lb. ground turkey
- 1 cup cauliflower rice
- 1 tsp garlic powder
- 1 tsp onion powder
- 2 cups no added sugar marinara sauce
- Salt and pepper to taste

Direction.

1. In a large bowl, combine ground turkey, cauliflower rice, garlic powder, onion powder, salt, and pepper. Form the mixture into 1-inch meatballs.
2. In a non-stick skillet over medium heat, add the marinara sauce and let it simmer.
3. Carefully place meatballs into the sauce and cover. Cook for 15 minutes, turning occasionally, until meatballs are cooked through.

Serving size: 3 meatballs with sauce

Tips: For extra flavor, add Italian seasoning / fresh herbs to the meat mixture.

Nutritional Values: Calories: 210; Carbs: 10g; Fat: 7g; Protein: 30g; Sugar: 4g; Sodium: 350mg; Fiber: 2g; Cholesterol: 90mg

84. Turkey Cauliflower Bake

Prep time: 10 min   Cook time: 15 min   Servings: 4

Ingredients:

- 1 lb. ground turkey
- 2 cups cauliflower florets
- 1 cup diced tomatoes (canned, no added salt)
- 1 tsp Italian seasoning
- 1/2 cup shredded low-fat cheese (optional)
- Salt and pepper to taste

Direction.

1. Preheat the oven to 375°F (190°C). In a large skillet over medium heat, cook ground turkey for 5 minutes until browned. Drain any excess fat.

2. Add cauliflower florets, tomatoes, Italian seasoning, salt, and pepper. Mix well.

3. Transfer the mixture to a baking dish and top with shredded cheese if desired. Bake for 15 minutes or until the cauliflower is tender.

Serving size: 1 cup

Tips: Feel free to add other zero-point veggies like spinach or bell peppers for additional nutrients.

Nutritional Values: Calories: 180; Carbs: 12g; Fat: 7g; Protein: 25g; Sugar: 2g; Sodium: 320mg; Fiber: 3g; Cholesterol: 70mg

CHAPTER 14

Meat Recipes

85.   Asian Beef Lettuce Wraps

Prep time: 10 min   Cook time: 15 min   Servings: 4

Ingredients:

- 1 lb. lean ground beef
- 1 cup mushrooms, finely chopped
- 1 cup shredded carrots
- ¼ cup low-sodium soy sauce
- 1 tbsp fresh ginger, grated
- 1 head butter or romaine lettuce, leaves separated

Direction.

1. In a skillet over medium heat, cook the ground beef until browned. Drain any excess fat.

2. Add the mushrooms, shredded carrots, soy sauce, and grated ginger. Stir well and cook for an additional 5-7 minutes until the vegetables are tender.

3. Remove and let cool slightly. Spoon the beef mixture into lettuce leaves and serve.

Serving size: 2 wraps

Tips: Serve with a side of sliced cucumbers for extra crunch.

Nutritional Values: Calories: 220; Carbs: 12g; Fat: 10g; Protein: 25g; Sugar: 2g; Sodium: 500mg; Fiber: 3g; Cholesterol: 75mg

86.   Beef and Mushroom Stroganoff

Prep time: 10 min   Cook time: 15 min   Servings: 4

Ingredients:

- 1 lb. lean ground beef
- 2 cups sliced mushrooms
- 1 cup onions, chopped
- 2 cups low-sodium beef broth
- 1 cup fat-free plain Greek yogurt
- 2 tsp garlic powder
- Salt and pepper to taste

Direction.

1. In a large skillet, brown the ground beef over medium heat for 5 minutes until fully cooked. Drain excess fat if necessary.

2. Add the onions and mushrooms, then sauté for 5 minutes until softened. Pour in the beef broth and simmer for another 5 minutes.

3. Reduce heat and stir in the Greek yogurt until blended. Season with garlic powder, salt, and pepper. Serve warm.

Serving size: 1 cup

Tips: Serve over whole grain pasta or zucchini noodles for added texture.

Nutritional Values: Calories: 230; Carbs: 8g; Fat: 10g; Protein: 28g; Sugar: 3g; Sodium: 450mg; Fiber: 1g; Cholesterol: 70mg

87.   Beefy Cauliflower Mash

Prep time: 5 min   Cook time: 15 min   Servings: 4

Ingredients:

- 1 lb. cauliflower florets
- 1 lb. lean ground beef
- 1/2 cup low-sodium beef broth
- 1/4 cup fat-free cream cheese
- 1 tsp onion powder
- Salt and pepper to taste

Direction.

1. Boil cauliflower florets in salted water for about 10 minutes or until tender. Drain and set aside.

2. In a skillet, cook the ground beef for 5 minutes over medium heat until browned. Drain any excess fat.

3. In a large bowl, combine the cauliflower, cooked beef, beef broth, and cream cheese. Mash until smooth. Stir in onion powder, salt, and pepper. Serve warm.

Serving size: 1 cup

Tips: Add a sprinkle of fresh herbs like parsley for extra flavor.

Nutritional Values: Calories: 200; Carbs: 6g; Fat: 9g; Protein: 25g; Sugar: 2g; Sodium: 350mg; Fiber: 2g; Cholesterol: 80mg

88.   Herb Garlic Grilled Flank Steak

Prep time: 10 min   Cook time: 10 min   Servings: 4

Ingredients:

- 1 lb. flank steak
- 2 tbsp minced garlic
- 2 tbsp chopped fresh parsley
- 1 tbsp chopped fresh rosemary
- 1 tsp black pepper
- Non-stick cooking spray

Direction.

1. Preheat your grill to medium-high heat.

2. In a small bowl, mix minced garlic, parsley, rosemary, and black pepper to create an herb paste.

3. Rub the herb mixture evenly over the flank steak.

4. Spray the grill with non-stick cooking spray to prevent sticking.

5. Grill the flank steak for about 5 minutes on each side.

6. Remove and let rest for a few minutes before slicing against the grain.

Serving size: 4 oz steak

Tips: Serve with a side of steamed vegetables for a complete meal.

Nutritional Values: Calories: 190; Carbs: 0g; Fat: 7g; Protein: 28g; Sugar: 0g; Sodium: 60mg; Fiber: 0g; Cholesterol: 70mg

89. Zucchini Noodles with Beef Bolognese

Prep time: 10 min   Cook time: 15 min   Servings: 4

Ingredients:

- 1 lb. lean ground beef (or turkey)
- 4 medium zucchinis, spiralized
- 1 cup no sugar added marinara sauce
- 1 tbsp Italian seasoning
- Salt and pepper to taste

Direction.

1. In a large skillet, brown the ground beef for 5-7 minutes over medium heat, breaking it apart until fully cooked. Drain any excess fat.

2. Add the marinara sauce, Italian seasoning, salt, and pepper to the skillet. Simmer for 5 minutes.

3. Meanwhile, add the zucchini to another skillet over medium heat and cook for 2-3 minutes until just tender.

4. Combine the zucchini noodles with the Bolognese sauce and toss to coat. Serve hot.

Serving size: 1 cup

Tips: For added flavor, sauté some garlic and onion in the skillet before adding the beef.

Nutritional Values: Calories: 230; Carbs: 6g; Fat: 11g; Protein: 26g; Sugar: 3g; Sodium: 400mg; Fiber: 2g; Cholesterol: 70mg

90. Pork and Cabbage Stir-Fry

Prep time: 10 min   Cook time: 15 min   Servings: 4

Ingredients:

- 1 lb. lean pork tenderloin, sliced thin
- 4 cups shredded green cabbage
- 1 cup sliced bell peppers (any color)
- 2 tbsp low-sodium soy sauce
- 1 tsp minced garlic
- Non-stick cooking spray

Direction.

1. Heat a large non-stick skillet over medium-high heat and spray with non-stick cooking spray.

2. Add the pork tenderloin to the skillet and cook for about 5-7 minutes, stirring occasionally, until browned.

3. Add the garlic and stir for 1 minute until fragrant.

4. Toss in the shredded cabbage and sliced bell peppers, stirring to combine.

5. Drizzle with soy sauce and cook for 5-7 minutes, until the vegetables are tender-crisp.

Serving size: 1 ½ cup

Tips: Serve over cauliflower rice for a low-carb meal.

Nutritional Values: Calories: 160; Carbs: 8g; Fat: 4g; Protein: 24g; Sugar: 2g; Sodium: 220mg; Fiber: 3g; Cholesterol: 70mg

91.   Crispy Baked Pork Tenderloin

Prep time: 10 min   Cook time: 15 min   Servings: 4

Ingredients:

- 1 lb. pork tenderloin
- 1 tsp olive oil
- 1 tsp garlic powder
- 1 tsp paprika
- 1 tsp black pepper
- 1 tsp onion powder
- ½ tsp salt

Direction.

1. Preheat your oven to 425°F (220°C).

2. In a small bowl, mix the olive oil, garlic powder, paprika, black pepper, onion powder, and salt.

3. Rub the spice mixture all over the pork tenderloin, ensuring it is evenly coated.

4. Place the pork tenderloin on a lined baking sheet.

5. Bake for 15 minutes or until the internal temperature reaches 145°F (63°C).

Serving Size: 4 oz (1/4 of the tenderloin)

Tips: Serve with steamed vegetables for a balanced meal. You can also use a meat thermometer for perfect doneness.

Nutritional Values: Calories: 150; Carbs: 0g; Fat: 3g; Protein: 26g; Sugar: 0g; Sodium: 300mg; Fiber: 0g; Cholesterol: 70mg

92.   Beefy Vegetable Chili

Prep time: 10 min   Cook time: 15 min   Servings: 4

Ingredients:

- 1 lb. lean ground beef (95% lean)
- 2 cups no salt added diced tomatoes (canned)
- 1 cup canned kidney beans, rinsed and drained
- 1 cup bell peppers, diced
- 1 cup onion, diced
- 1 tbsp chili powder

Direction.

1. In a large pot over medium heat, brown the ground beef until fully cooked. Drain any excess fat. Add the onion and bell peppers to the pot, and sauté for 3-4 minutes until softened.

2. Stir in the diced tomatoes, kidney beans, and chili powder. Bring to a simmer. Cover & cook for an additional 10 minutes, stirring occasionally.

3. Season with salt and pepper as desired. Serve.

Serving size: 1 cup

Tips: Add some jalapeños for a spicy kick or top with fresh cilantro for extra flavor!

Nutritional Values: Calories: 250; Carbs: 28g; Fat: 8g; Protein: 22g; Sugar: 3g; Sodium: 200mg; Fiber: 7g; Cholesterol: 70mg

93. Sweet and Sour Pork with Bell Peppers

Prep time: 10 min   Cook time: 15 min   Servings: 4

Ingredients:

• 1 lb. lean pork tenderloin, cut into bite-sized pieces

• 1 cup bell peppers, sliced

• 1 cup fresh pineapple chunks (or canned in juice), drained

• 1/4 cup low-sodium soy sauce

• 2 tbsp rice vinegar

• 2 tbsp zero-calorie sweetener (like Stevia or Monk Fruit)

Direction.

1. In a large skillet, heat a non-stick pan over medium-high heat. Add the pork pieces and cook for 5-7 minutes until browned.

2. Add the bell peppers and pineapple chunks, then cook for another 3-4 minutes until peppers are slightly tender.

3. In a small bowl, mix the soy sauce, rice vinegar, and sweetener. Pour this mixture over the pork and vegetables.

4. Cook for an additional 5 minutes, allowing the sauce to thicken slightly. Stir occasionally. Serve warm.

Serving size: 1 cup

Tips: Serve over cauliflower rice for a healthy, low-carb option!

Nutritional Values: Calories: 220; Carbs: 24g; Fat: 5g; Protein: 24g; Sugar: 9g; Sodium: 480mg; Fiber: 2g; Cholesterol: 70mg

94. Beef and Zucchini Casserole

Prep time: 10 min   Cook time: 12 min   Servings: 4

Ingredients:

• 1 lb. lean ground beef

• 2 cups zucchini, sliced

• 1 cup low-sugar marinara sauce

• 1 cup shredded low-fat mozzarella cheese

• 1 tsp Italian seasoning

• Salt and pepper to taste

Direction.

1. Preheat your oven to 375°F (190°C). In a skillet over medium heat, cook the ground beef for 5-7 minutes until browned. Drain excess fat if necessary.

2. Add the zucchini, marinara sauce, Italian seasoning, salt, and pepper. Stir well to combine and cook for an additional 5 minutes.

3. Transfer the mixture to a baking dish and top with mozzarella cheese. Bake for 15 minutes, or until the cheese is melted. Serve.

Serving size: 1 cup

Tips: Pair with a side salad for a refreshing crunch.

Nutritional Values: Calories: 220; Carbs: 8g; Fat: 12g; Protein: 24g; Sugar: 4g; Sodium: 350mg; Fiber: 1g; Cholesterol: 70mg

95. Spiced Pork Tenderloin

Prep time: 5 min   Cook time: 20 min   Servings: 4

Ingredients:

- 1 lb. pork tenderloin
- 1 tsp garlic powder
- 1 tsp paprika
- 1 tsp ground cumin
- Salt and pepper to taste
- Non-stick cooking spray

Direction.

1. Preheat a non-stick skillet over medium-high heat and spray with non-stick cooking spray. Season the pork tenderloin with garlic powder, paprika, cumin, salt, and pepper.

2. Sear the pork on all sides for 3-4 minutes until browned. Adjust to medium, cover, and cook for an additional 15 minutes. Remove, let rest for 5 minutes, then slice and serve.

Serving size: 4 ounces

Tips: Leftovers can be used in salads or wraps.

Nutritional Values: Calories: 160; Carbs: 1g; Fat: 3g; Protein: 24g; Sugar: 0g; Sodium: 70mg; Fiber: 0g; Cholesterol: 70mg

96. Pork and Apple Skewers

Prep time: 10 min   Cook time: 15 min   Servings: 4

Ingredients:

- 1 lb. pork tenderloin, cut into 1-inch cubes
- 2 cups apple chunks (preferably firm apples like Granny Smith)
- 1 tbsp balsamic vinegar
- 1 tsp dried thyme
- 1 tsp onion powder
- Salt and pepper to taste

Direction.

1. Preheat the grill over medium-high heat. In a bowl, combine the pork cubes, apple chunks, balsamic vinegar, thyme, onion powder, salt, and pepper.

2. Thread the pork and apple pieces onto skewers, alternating them. Grill the skewers for about 10-12 minutes, turning occasionally, until the pork has nice grill marks.

Serving size: 2 skewers

Tips: Serve with a side of mixed greens for a refreshing meal.

Nutritional Values: Calories: 180; Carbs: 7g; Fat: 4g; Protein: 28g; Sugar: 3g; Sodium: 80mg; Fiber: 1g; Cholesterol: 75mg

CHAPTER 15
Vegetable Recipes

97.   Pumpkin and Black Bean Chili

 Prep time: 10 min   Cook time: 12 min   Servings: 4

Ingredients:

- 2 cups canned pumpkin puree
- 1 can (15 oz) black beans, drained and rinsed
- 1 cup vegetable broth
- 1 cup diced tomatoes
- 1 cup corn (frozen or canned)
- 1 tbsp chili powder

Direction.

1. In a large pot, combine the pumpkin puree, black beans, vegetable broth, diced tomatoes, corn, and chili powder.

2. Let it simmer over medium heat for about 15 minutes, stirring occasionally Adjust seasoning with salt and pepper as desired.

Serving size: 1 cup

Tips: Top with fresh cilantro or avocado for extra flavor!

Nutritional Values: Calories: 150; Carbs: 28g; Fat: 1g; Protein: 7g; Sugar: 4g; Sodium: 300mg; Fiber: 7g; Cholesterol: 0mg

98.   Vegetable Ratatouille

 Prep time: 10 min   Cook time: 12 min   Servings: 4

Ingredients:

- 1 medium zucchini, diced
- 1 medium eggplant, diced
- 1 bell pepper, diced
- 1 cup cherry tomatoes, halved
- 1/2 onion, diced
- Non-stick cooking spray

Direction.

1. Spray a large skillet with non-stick cooking spray and heat over medium heat. Add the onion and sauté for 2-3 minutes until translucent.

2. Add the zucchini, eggplant, and bell pepper, then cook for another 5 minutes until slightly tender.

3. Stir in the cherry tomatoes and cook for an additional 5-7 minutes, until all vegetables are soft. Season with salt, pepper, and herbs as desired.

Serving size: 1 cup

Tips: For added flavor, incorporate fresh herbs like parsley or thyme if you have them on hand.

Nutritional Values: Calories: 80; Carbs: 18g; Fat: 0g; Protein: 3g; Sugar: 4g; Sodium: 25mg; Fiber: 5g; Cholesterol: 0mg

99.   Broccoli and Cauliflower Bake

Prep time: 10 min   Cook time: 12 min   Servings: 4

Ingredients:

- 4 cups broccoli florets
- 4 cups cauliflower florets
- 1 cup low-sodium vegetable broth
- 1 tsp garlic powder
- 1 tsp onion powder
- 1 cup nutritional yeast

Direction.

1. Preheat your oven to 400°F (200°C). In a large pot, let the broth boil and add the broccoli and cauliflower. Cook for 3-5 minutes until slightly tender, then drain.

2. In a mixing bowl, combine the garlic powder, onion powder, and nutritional yeast. Place the cooked broccoli and cauliflower in a baking dish, sprinkle the seasoning mixture evenly over the top, and toss to coat.

3. Bake for 10-12 minutes until heated through and slightly golden.

Serving size: 1 cup

Tips: Add your favorite herbs for extra flavor!

Nutritional Values: Calories: 100; Carbs: 15g; Fat: 2g; Protein: 6g; Sugar: 2g; Sodium: 150mg; Fiber: 5g; Cholesterol: 0mg

100.   Zucchini Noodles with Avocado Pesto

Prep time: 10 min   Cook time: 5 min   Servings: 2

Ingredients:

- 4 cups zucchini noodles, spiralized
- 1 ripe avocado, medium
- 2 tbsp lemon juice
- 1 clove garlic, minced
- 1/4 cup fresh basil leaves
- Salt and pepper to taste

Direction.

1. In a blender or food processor, combine avocado, lemon juice, garlic, basil, salt, and pepper. Blend until smooth and creamy.

2. In a large skillet over medium heat, add zucchini noodles and sauté for 2-3 minutes until slightly softened. Remove and mix in the avocado pesto until thoroughly combined.

Serving size: 2 cups

Tips: Top with cherry tomatoes for added color and flavor!

Nutritional Values: Calories: 180; Carbs: 14g; Fat: 12g; Protein: 4g; Sugar: 1g; Sodium: 200mg; Fiber: 6g; Cholesterol: 0mg

101. Vegetable Sushi Rolls

Prep time: 15 min   Cook time: 10 min   Servings: 2

Ingredients:

- 1 cup sushi rice, rinsed
- 1 ½ cups water
- ½ cup cucumber, julienned
- ½ cup carrot, julienned
- ½ avocado, sliced
- 4 sheets nori (seaweed)

Direction.

1. Combine sushi rice with water in a medium saucepan and bring to a boil. Adjust to low, cover, and simmer for 10 minutes until rice is tender.

2. Let the rice cool slightly, then lay out a sheet of nori on a clean surface. Spread about ¼ cup of rice evenly over the nori, leaving a 1-inch border at the top.

3. Arrange a few pieces of cucumber, carrot, and avocado in a line along the bottom edge of the rice.

4. Roll the sushi tightly from the bottom up, using the mat to help. Seal the edge with a little water.

5. Repeat with remaining nori and fillings. Slice each roll into bite-sized pieces.

Serving size: 4 pieces

Tips: Serve with low-sodium soy sauce or pickled ginger for an extra flavor kick!

Nutritional Values: Calories: 300; Carbs: 64g; Fat: 7g; Protein: 8g; Sugar: 2g; Sodium: 10mg; Fiber: 6g; Cholesterol: 0mg

102. Vegetable Soba Noodles Bowl

Prep time: 10 min   Cook time: 15 min   Servings: 2

Ingredients:

- 7 oz soba noodles
- 1 cup broccoli florets
- ½ cup bell pepper, sliced
- ½ cup snap peas
- 2 tbsp low-sodium soy sauce
- 1 tbsp sesame seeds (optional)

Direction.

1. Cook the soba noodles according to package instructions. Drain & set aside.

2. In a large skillet, bring a small amount of water to a boil. Add broccoli, bell pepper, and snap peas, and steam for about 4-5 minutes until tender but crisp.

3. Add the cooked soba noodles with the steamed vegetables. Pour in the soy sauce and toss to combine.

4. Cook for an additional 2-3 minutes until heated through. Sprinkle with sesame seeds before serving, if desired.

Serving size: 1 bowl

Tips: Add your favorite spices or a splash of rice vinegar for extra flavor!

Nutritional Values: Calories: 220; Carbs: 45g; Fat: 3g; Protein: 9g; Sugar: 2g; Sodium: 200mg; Fiber: 5g; Cholesterol: 0mg

103. Cauliflower Steaks with Chimichurri

Prep time: 10 min | **Cook time:** 15 min | **Servings:** 2

Ingredients:

- 1 head cauliflower (about 1 lb.)
- 1 cup fresh parsley, chopped
- 1 tbsp red wine vinegar
- 1 tsp garlic, minced
- 1 tsp red pepper flakes
- Non-stick cooking spray

Direction.

1. Preheat a grill pan or oven to medium-high heat.
2. Slice the cauliflower head into 1-inch thick steaks.
3. Spray the grill pan with non-stick cooking spray and place the cauliflower steaks on it. Cook for 5-7 minutes on each side until tender and slightly charred.
4. In a small bowl, mix the parsley, red wine vinegar, garlic, and red pepper flakes to create the chimichurri sauce.
5. Serve the cauliflower steaks drizzled with chimichurri sauce.

Serving size: 1 steak with chimichurri

Tips: For added flavor, let the chimichurri sit for a few minutes before serving.

Nutritional Values: Calories: 80; Carbs: 9g; Fat: 2g; Protein: 4g; Sugar: 1g; Sodium: 75mg; Fiber: 4g; Cholesterol: 0mg

104. Asparagus & Lemon Quinoa

Prep time: 10 min | **Cook time:** 15 min | **Servings:** 4

Ingredients:

- 1 cup quinoa, rinsed
- 2 cups low sodium vegetable broth
- 1 lb. fresh asparagus, trimmed and cut into 2-inch pieces
- 1 lemon, zested and juiced
- 1 tsp garlic powder
- Non-stick cooking spray

Direction.

1. In a medium saucepan, combine quinoa and broth. Let it boil, cover, and simmer for 15 minutes or until quinoa is fluffy.
2. Meanwhile, spray a non-stick skillet with cooking spray and add asparagus. Sauté over medium heat for about 5-7 minutes until tender.
3. Once the quinoa is cooked, fluff it with a fork and stir in lemon juice, lemon zest, garlic powder, and sautéed asparagus.
4. Mix well and season with salt and pepper. Serve warm.

Serving size: 1/2 cup quinoa mixture

Tips: For a little extra crunch, toast the quinoa in the pot for a few minutes before adding the broth.

Nutritional Values: Calories: 150; Carbs: 30g; Fat: 1g; Protein: 5g; Sugar: 1g; Sodium: 200mg; Fiber: 4g; Cholesterol: 0mg

105. Vegetable Paella

Prep time: 10 min   Cook time: 15 min   Servings: 4

Ingredients:

- 2 cups cauliflower rice
- 1 cup red bell pepper, diced
- 1 cup green peas (fresh/ frozen)
- 1 cup diced tomatoes (canned, no salt added)
- 1 cup low-sodium vegetable broth
- 1 tsp smoked paprika
- Salt and pepper to taste
- Non-stick cooking spray

Direction.

1. Spray a large non-stick skillet with cooking spray & heat over medium-high heat.
2. Add the red bell pepper and sauté for 2-3 mins until slightly softened.
3. Stir in the cauliflower rice, diced tomatoes, green peas, and broth.
4. Add the smoked paprika, salt, and pepper, stirring to combine.
5. Cover and simmer for 10 mins, allowing the vegetables to cook through.

Serving size: 1 cup

Tips: Serve with a sprinkle of fresh parsley or lemon juice for extra flavor.

Nutritional Values: Calories: 80; Carbs: 15g; Fat: 0g; Protein: 4g; Sugar: 3g; Sodium: 200mg; Fiber: 4g; Cholesterol: 0mg

106. Vegan Eggplant Lasagna

Prep time: 10 min   Cook time: 20 min   Servings: 4

Ingredients:

- 2 medium eggplants (sliced into ¼-inch rounds)
- 2 cups of marinara sauce (sugar-free)
- 1 cup of spinach (fresh or frozen)
- 1 cup of mushrooms, sliced
- 1 tsp of garlic powder
- 1 tsp of Italian seasoning

Direction.

1. Preheat your oven to 375°F (190°C).
2. Spray a baking dish with non-stick cooking spray and layer half of the eggplant slices on the bottom.
3. Spread half of the marinara sauce over the eggplant, followed by half of the spinach and mushrooms.
4. Sprinkle garlic powder and Italian seasoning over the top.
5. Repeat the layers with the remaining eggplant, marinara sauce, spinach, & mushrooms.
6. Cover with foil and bake for 15 minutes, removing the foil for the last 5 minutes to allow the top to brown slightly.

Serving size: 1/4 of the dish

Tips: Let the lasagna sit for a few minutes before cutting for cleaner slices.

Nutritional Values: Calories: 130; Carbs: 16g; Fat: 1g; Protein: 4g; Sugar: 3g; Sodium: 200mg; Fiber: 6g; Cholesterol: 0mg

107. Mediterranean Stuffed Eggplant

Prep time: 10 min   Cook time: 15 min   Servings: 4

Ingredients:

- 1 medium eggplant
- 1 cup diced tomatoes (canned or fresh)
- 1 cup chopped bell pepper
- 1 cup cooked lentils (canned or fresh)
- 1 tsp garlic powder
- 1 tsp Italian seasoning
- Non-stick cooking spray

Direction.

1. Preheat your oven to 400°F (200°C).
2. Slice the eggplant in half lengthwise and scoop out some of the flesh to create a boat.
3. In a bowl, mix tomatoes, bell pepper, lentils, garlic powder, & Italian seasoning.
4. Fill the eggplant halves with the mixture and place them on a baking sheet sprayed with cooking spray.
5. Bake for about 15 minutes, or until the eggplant is tender.

Serving size: 1 stuffed eggplant half

Tips: You can customize your filling by adding other zero-point vegetables like zucchini or mushrooms.

Nutritional Values: Calories: 120; Carbs: 26g; Fat: 0.5g; Protein: 5g; Sugar: 4g; Sodium: 150mg; Fiber: 10g; Cholesterol: 0mg

108. Vegetable Stir-Fried Cauliflower Rice

Prep time: 10 min   Cook time: 15 min   Servings: 4

Ingredients:

- 4 cups cauliflower rice (fresh or frozen)
- 1 cup bell peppers, diced
- 1 cup broccoli florets
- 1 cup carrots, shredded
- 1 tsp garlic powder
- 1 tbsp soy sauce (low-sodium or sugar-free)

Direction.

1. Spray a large non-stick skillet with non-stick cooking spray and heat over medium-high.
2. Add the bell peppers, broccoli, and carrots. Stir-fry for 5-7 mins until tender.
3. Stir in the cauliflower rice, garlic powder, & soy sauce, mixing well to combine.
4. Cook for an additional 5-7 minutes, stirring occasionally, until the cauliflower is heated through. Serve.

Serving size: 1 cup

Tips: Garnish with chopped green onions for added freshness.

Nutritional Values: Calories: 50; Carbs: 10g; Fat: 0g; Protein: 4g; Sugar: 3g; Sodium: 220mg; Fiber: 4g; Cholesterol: 0mg

CHAPTER 16
Refreshing Desserts

109. Matcha Green Tea Yogurt Cups

 Prep time: 10 min   Cook time: 0 min   Servings: 4 Cup

Ingredients:

• 2 cups non-fat Greek yogurt or silken tofu

• 1/4 cup matcha green tea powder

• 1/2 cup sugar-free sweetener (like Stevia or Erythritol)

• 1 tbsp lemon juice

• Fresh berries for garnish (optional)

Direction.

1. In a mixing bowl, combine the non-fat Greek yogurt, matcha green tea powder, sweetener, and lemon juice.

2. Whisk together until smooth and creamy.

3. Spoon the mixture into small serving cups or glasses.

4. Chill in the refrigerator for at least 15 minutes before serving.

5. Top with fresh berries if desired.

Serving size: 1 cup

Tips: Prepare the cups in advance for a quick grab-and-go dessert.

Nutritional Values: Calories: 90; Carbs: 8g; Fat: 0g; Protein: 9g; Sugar: 2g; Sodium: 50mg; Fiber: 1g; Cholesterol: 0mg

110. Spiced Baked Apples

 Prep time: 5 min   Cook time: 20 min   Servings: 4

Ingredients:

• 4 medium apples, cored and sliced

• 1 tsp cinnamon

• 1/2 tsp nutmeg

• 1/4 cup sugar-free sweetener (like Stevia or Erythritol)

• 1 tbsp lemon juice

• 1/2 cup water

Direction.

1. Preheat the oven to 350°F (175°C).

2. In a large baking dish, combine the sliced apples, cinnamon, nutmeg, sugar-free sweetener, lemon juice, and water.

3. Cover with aluminum foil and bake for 20 mins, or until apples are tender.

Serving size: 1 apple (about 1/2 cup)

Tips: Serve with a dollop of non-fat Greek yogurt for added creaminess.

Nutritional Values: Calories: 60; Carbs: 16g; Fat: 0g; Protein: 0g; Sugar: 4g; Sodium: 0mg; Fiber: 3g; Cholesterol: 0mg

111. Lemon Basil Sorbet

Prep time: 10 minutes + chilling time **Cook time: 15 min** **Servings: 4**

Ingredients:

- 2 cups water
- 1 cup fresh lemon juice
- 1/2 cup sugar-free sweetener (like Stevia or Erythritol)
- 1/2 cup fresh basil leaves, chopped
- Pinch of salt
- Lemon zest for garnish (optional)

Direction.

1. In a saucepan, combine water, lemon juice, and sugar-free sweetener. Heat over medium, stirring occasionally.

2. Remove & stir in the chopped basil and salt. Allow it to cool for about 5 mins.

3. Pour the mixture into a shallow dish and freeze, stirring every 30 mins.

4. Serve immediately. Garnish with lemon zest if desired.

Serving size: 1/2 cup

Tips: Serve with fresh basil leaves or lemon slices for a refreshing presentation!

Nutritional Values: Calories: 35; Carbs: 9g; Fat: 0g; Protein: 0g; Sugar: 0g; Sodium: 5mg; Fiber: 0g; Cholesterol: 0mg

112. Sweet Potato Brownies

Prep time: 10 min **Cook time: 15 min** **Servings: 8**

Ingredients:

- 1 cup cooked sweet potato, mashed
- 1 cup rolled oats (blended into oat flour)
- 1/2 cup unsweetened applesauce
- 1/4 cup sugar-free sweetener (like Stevia or erythritol)
- 1/4 cup unsweetened almond milk
- 1/2 tsp baking powder

Direction.

1. Preheat your oven to 350°F (175°C) and lightly grease an 8-inch square baking dish.

2. In a large bowl, combine the mashed sweet potato, oat flour, applesauce, sweetener, almond milk, and baking powder.

3. Pour the batter into the prepared baking dish and spread evenly.

4. Bake for 15 minutes or until a toothpick inserted in the center comes out clean.

5. Let the brownies cool for a few mins before cutting into squares & serving.

Serving size: 1 brownie

Tips: For an extra touch, top with a sprinkle of cinnamon before baking.

Nutritional Values: Calories: 90; Carbs: 19g; Fat: 0.5g; Protein: 3g; Sugar: 2g; Sodium: 5mg; Fiber: 2g; Cholesterol: 0mg

113. Ginger-Spiced Pear Crisp

Prep time: 10 min   Cook time: 15 min   Servings: 4

Ingredients:

- 4 cups sliced pears
- 1 tsp ground ginger
- 1 tsp cinnamon
- 1 tbsp lemon juice
- 1 tbsp sugar-free sweetener (like Stevia or erythritol)
- 1/2 tsp salt

Direction.

1. Preheat your oven to 350°F (175°C).

2. In a bowl, mix pears, ginger, cinnamon, lemon juice, sweetener, and salt.

3. Transfer the mixture to a baking dish and spread evenly.

4. Bake for 15 minutes or until the mixture is bubbly. Serve warm.

Serving size: 1 cup

Tips: Top with a dollop of nonfat Greek yogurt for added flavor without the points!

Nutritional Values: Calories: 120; Carbs: 28g; Fat: 0g; Protein: 1g; Sugar: 8g; Sodium: 50mg; Fiber: 4g; Cholesterol: 0mg

114. Creamy Pineapple Popsicles

Prep time: 5 minutes + freezing time   Cook time: 0 min   Servings: 6

Ingredients:

- 2 cups unsweetened almond milk (or a mix of coconut water and non-fat Greek yogurt)
- 1 cup fresh pineapple chunks
- 1 tsp vanilla extract
- 1 cup blueberries
- Pinch of salt

Direction.

1. In a blender, combine unsweetened almond milk, pineapple chunks, vanilla extract, and salt. Blend until smooth.

2. Divide the mixture evenly among popsicle molds, filling them halfway. Add a few blueberries into each mold and top off with the remaining coconut mixture.

3. Insert popsicle sticks and freeze for at least 4 hours or until solid. To release the popsicles, run warm water over the outside of the molds for a few seconds.

Serving size: 1 popsicle

Tips: Experiment with other fruits like mango or strawberries for variety!

Nutritional Values: Calories: 25; Carbs: 8g; Fat: 0.5g; Protein: 1g; Sugar: 4g; Sodium: 20mg; Fiber: 1g; Cholesterol: 0mg

115. Carrot Cake Energy Bites

Prep time: 10 min   **Cook time: 0 min**   **Servings: 12 bites**

Ingredients:

- 1 cup grated carrots
- 1/2 cup unsweetened applesauce
- 1/2 cup crushed almonds (portion-controlled)
- 1 tsp cinnamon
- 1 tsp sugar-free syrup (optional)

Direction.

1. In a large bowl, combine grated carrots, applesauce, crushed almonds, cinnamon, and sugar-free syrup (if using). Mix until well combined.

2. Use your hands to form the mixture into small balls. Place the energy bites on a lined baking sheet. Refrigerate for at least 15 minutes to firm them up.

Serving size: 1 energy bite

Tips: You can add a pinch of nutmeg or ginger for extra flavor.

Nutritional Values: Calories: 40; Carbs: 5g; Fat: 1.5g; Protein: 1g; Sugar: 2g; Sodium: 1mg; Fiber: 1g; Cholesterol: 0mg

116. Raspberry Chia Jam

Prep time: 15 min   **Cook time: 0 min**   **Servings: 8**

Ingredients:

- 2 cups fresh or frozen raspberries
- 2 tbsp chia seeds
- 1 tbsp lemon juice
- 1/2 tsp vanilla extract
- Pinch of salt

Direction.

1. In a medium bowl, mash the raspberries until they reach your desired consistency.

2. Stir in the chia seeds, lemon juice, vanilla extract, and salt until blended.

3. Let the mixture sit for about 10-15 minutes to thicken. Transfer to a clean jar and refrigerate for up to 2 weeks.

Serving size: 2 tbsp

Tips: This jam is perfect for spreading on toast or adding to yogurt. Feel free to experiment with other fruits!

Nutritional Values: Calories: 30; Carbs: 7g; Fat: 1g; Protein: 1g; Sugar: 3g; Sodium: 5mg; Fiber: 3g; Cholesterol: 0mg

117. Pumpkin Spice Muffins

Prep time: 10 min   Cook time: 15 min   Servings: 12

Ingredients:

- 1 cup canned pumpkin puree
- 1/2 cup oat flour made from zero-point oats (optional: finely ground zero-point oats in a blender)
- 1/2 cup unsweetened applesauce
- 1 tsp pumpkin pie spice
- 1 tsp baking powder

Direction.

1. Preheat the oven to 350°F (175°C) and line a muffin tin with paper liners.

2. In a large bowl, mix pumpkin puree, oat flour, applesauce, pumpkin pie spice, and baking powder.

3. Pour the batter into the prepared muffin tin. Bake for 15 minutes or until a toothpick inserted in the center comes out clean.

Serving size: 1 muffin

Tips: You can add chopped walnuts or dried cranberries for added texture and flavor, but be mindful of the portion to keep it zero point.

Nutritional Values: Calories: 40; Carbs: 9g; Fat: 0.5g; Protein: 1g; Sugar: 3g; Sodium: 15mg; Fiber: 2g; Cholesterol: 0mg

118. Classic Fruit Salad

Prep time: 10 min   Cook time: 0 min   Servings: 4

Ingredients:

- 2 cups diced watermelon
- 1 cup diced pineapple
- 1 cup sliced strawberries
- 1 cup blueberries
- 1 tbsp lime juice

Direction.

1. In a large bowl, combine the watermelon, pineapple, strawberries, and blueberries.

2. Drizzle the lime juice over the fruit and gently toss to combine. Serve.

Serving size: 1 cup

Tips: Feel free to mix in any seasonal fruits you have on hand for variety!

Nutritional Values: Calories: 40; Carbs: 15g; Fat: 0g; Protein: 1g; Sugar: 5g; Sodium: 5mg; Fiber: 2g; Cholesterol: 0mg

119. Frozen Candy Grapes

Prep time: 10 minutes + freezing time **Cook time: 0 min** **Servings: 4**

Ingredients:

- 2 cups seedless grapes (any variety)
- 1 cup sugar-free nonfat Greek yogurt
- 1/4 cup sugar-free sweetener (like Stevia or erythritol)
- 1/2 tsp lemon juice
- Pinch of salt

Direction.

1. Wash the grapes thoroughly and pat them dry with a paper towel.
2. In a mixing bowl, combine the yogurt, sweetener, lemon juice, and salt. Stir until well mixed.
3. Dip each grape in the yogurt mixture, ensuring they are fully coated.
4. Place the coated grapes on a lined baking sheet in a single layer.
5. Freeze for at least 2 hours until completely solid.
6. Enjoy your frozen candy grapes straight from the freezer!

Serving size: 1 cup

Tips: For added flavor, experiment with different yogurt flavors or add spices like cinnamon.

Nutritional Values: Calories: 80; Carbs: 17g; Fat: 0g; Protein: 2g; Sugar: 9g; Sodium: 20mg; Fiber: 1g; Cholesterol: 0mg

120. Cinnamon Stewed Pears

Prep time: 10 min **Cook time: 15 min** **Servings: 4**

Ingredients:

- 4 ripe pears, peeled and sliced
- 1/4 cup water
- 1 tsp ground cinnamon
- 1 tsp vanilla extract
- 1 tbsp lemon juice

Direction.

1. In a medium saucepan, mix pears, water, cinnamon, vanilla, and lemon juice.
2. Cook over medium heat for about 15-20 minutes, stirring occasionally, until the pears are tender. Remove and let cool slightly before serving.

Serving size: 1 cup

Tips: Serve warm or chilled, and for an extra treat, add a dollop of yogurt on top.

Nutritional Values: Calories: 60; Carbs: 15g; Fat: 0g; Protein: 1g; Sugar: 10g; Sodium: 0mg; Fiber: 3g; Cholesterol: 0mg

30-DAY MEAL PLAN

DAY	BREAKFAST	LUNCH	SNACKS/DESSERT	DINNER
1	Zucchini & Tomato Egg Bake	Savory Chicken and Mushroom Skillet	Matcha Green Tea Yogurt Cups	Pumpkin and Black Bean Chili
2	Cauliflower Hash Browns	Chili Lime Grilled Shrimp Tacos	Watermelon Cucumber Gazpacho Shooters	Broccoli and Cauliflower Bake
3	Zero Breakfast Energy Bites	Black Bean Lentil Burgers	Cinnamon Stewed Pears	Asian Beef Lettuce Wraps
4	Mushroom & Spinach Scramble	Turkey Cauliflower Bake	Jicama Sticks with Lime	Vegetable Stir-Fried Cauliflower Rice
5	Carrot Cake Overnight Oats	Teriyaki Glazed Mahi Mahi	Frozen Candy Grapes	Egg Drop Soup with Chicken
6	Turnip Breakfast Bowl with Herbs	Cauliflower Rice with Grilled Chicken Bowl	Herbed Cauliflower Cakes	Pork and Apple Skewers
7	Savory Cauliflower Porridge	Turkey Meatballs with Marinara	Classic Fruit Salad	Mediterranean Stuffed Eggplant
8	Cauliflower Rice Breakfast Bowl	Grilled Swordfish with Mango Salsa	Spicy Roasted Chickpeas	Light Dahl with Spinach
9	Berry Blast Yogurt Parfait	Zucchini Noodles with Broccoli Rabe	Pumpkin Spice Muffins	Blackened Catfish with Cabbage Slaw
10	Cheesy Spinach and Egg Bake	Miso Glazed Chicken Thighs	Tuna Celery Boats	Vegan Eggplant Lasagna
11	Apple & Cinnamon Yogurt Bowl	Coconut Curry Lobster	Raspberry Chia Jam	Beef and Zucchini Casserole
12	Bell Pepper & Onion Frittata	Spaghetti Squash Primavera	Cucumber Rounds with Zero-Point Hummus	Garlic and Rosemary Roast Turkey Breast
13	Breakfast Stuffed Spaghetti Squash	Glazed Garlic Chicken Drumsticks	Carrot Cake Energy Bites	Vegetable Paella
14	Pumpkin Spice Oatmeal	Sautéed Scallops with Asparagus	Tomato Basil Bruschetta	Crispy Baked Pork Tenderloin
15	Zucchini Bread Muffins	Cauliflower Gnocchi in Tomato Basil Sauce	Spiced Baked Apples	Vegetable Ratatouille

16	Berry Chia Seed Smoothie Bowl	Turkey and Quinoa Stuffed Zucchini	Cauliflower Buffalo Bites	Garlic Lemon Prawns with Quinoa
17	Peach & Ginger Yogurt Cup	Baked Halibut with Tomato Basil Relish	Coconut Milk Popsicles	Cauliflower Rice with Grilled Veggies
18	Egg White Omelet with Salsa	Bulgur Wheat Tacos	Vegetable Crudité Platter	Asparagus & Lemon Quinoa
19	Egg White Breakfast Burrito	Turkey Cabbage Roll Casserole	Ginger-Spiced Pear Crisp	Sweet and Sour Pork with Bell Peppers
20	Banana Oatmeal Muffins	Baked Salmon with Dill Yogurt Sauce	Baked Kale Chips	Moroccan Carrot and Chickpea Stew
21	Zucchini & Tomato Egg Bake	Beefy Cauliflower Mash	Lemon Basil Sorbet	Cauliflower Steaks with Chimichurri
22	Cauliflower Hash Browns	Chickpea and Cauliflower Rice Buddha Bowl	Spicy Roasted Chickpeas	Herbed Chicken Quinoa Bowl
23	Zero Breakfast Energy Bites	Seafood Chowder with Cauliflower Base	Sweet Potato Brownies	Beefy Vegetable Chili
24	Mushroom & Spinach Scramble	Herb Garlic Grilled Flank Steak	Matcha Green Tea Yogurt Cups	Vegetable Soba Noodles Bowl
25	Carrot Cake Overnight Oats	Lentil Salad with Roasted Vegetables	Watermelon Cucumber Gazpacho Shooters	Fish Tandoori Skewers
26	Turnip Breakfast Bowl with Herbs	Sardine and Avocado Salad	Cinnamon Stewed Pears	Beef and Mushroom Stroganoff
27	Savory Cauliflower Porridge	Zucchini Noodles with Beef Bolognese	Jicama Sticks with Lime	Vegetable Sushi Rolls
28	Cauliflower Rice Breakfast Bowl	Cauliflower Rice and Beans Stuffed Peppers	Frozen Candy Grapes	Mediterranean Chicken Skewers
29	Berry Blast Yogurt Parfait	Buffalo Chicken Lettuce Wraps	Herbed Cauliflower Cakes	Spiced Pork Tenderloin
30	Cheesy Spinach and Egg Bake	Pork and Cabbage Stir-Fry	Classic Fruit Salad	Zucchini Noodles with Avocado Pesto

FULL ZERO POINT FOODS LIST

FRUITS

- Apples
- Applesauce, unsweetened
- Apricots, fresh
- Bananas
- Blackberries
- Blueberries
- Cantaloupes
- Cherries
- Clementines
- Cranberries, fresh
- Dragon fruit
- Figs, fresh
- Fruit cocktail, unsweetened
- Fruit salad, unsweetened
- Frozen mixed berries, unsweetened
- Fruit, canned in water with or without artificial sweeteners
- Grapefruit
- Grapes
- Guavas
- Honeydew melons
- Jackfruit
- Kiwis
- Kumquats
- Lemons
- Limes
- Mangoes
- Meyer lemons
- Nectarines
- Oranges
- Papayas
- Peaches
- Pears
- Persimmons
- Pineapples
- Plums
- Pomegranates
- Pomelos
- Raspberries
- Star fruit
- Strawberries
- Tangerines
- Watermelons

NON-STARCHY VEGETABLES

- Artichoke hearts, without oil
- Arugula
- Asparagus
- Baby corn
- Bamboo shoots
- Beet greens
- Beets
- Bell peppers
- Bok choy
- Broccoli
- Broccoli rabe
- Broccoli slaw
- Brussels sprouts
- Butter lettuce (Bibb or Boston)
- Butternut squash
- Cabbage
- Carrots
- Cauliflower
- Cauliflower rice
- Celery
- Chiles
- Coleslaw mix
- Collard greens
- Cucumbers
- Delicata squash
- Eggplants
- Endive
- Escarole
- Fennel
- Frozen stir-fry vegetables, without sauce
- Frozen vegetable mixes
- Green beans
- Green leaf lettuce
- Hearts of palm
- Iceberg lettuce
- Jalapeño peppers
- Jicama
- Kale
- Kohlrabi
- Leeks
- Mixed greens
- Mushrooms
- Mustard greens
- Napa cabbage
- Nori (dried seaweed)
- Oak leaf lettuce
- Okra
- Onions
- Pea shoots
- Pickles, unsweetened
- Pico de gallo
- Pimientos, canned
- Pumpkin
- Pumpkin purée
- Radishes
- Red leaf lettuce
- Romaine lettuce
- Rutabaga
- Salsa, fat-free
- Sauerkraut
- Scallions
- Shallots
- Snow peas
- Spaghetti squash
- Spinach
- Summer squash
- Sugar snap peas
- Swiss chard
- Tomatillos
- Tomato purée, canned
- Tomatoes
- Turnips
- Water chestnuts
- Wax beans
- Zucchini

CHICKEN & TURKEY

- Chicken breast, skinless
- Chicken, canned in water
- Ground chicken breast
- Ground chicken, 90% lean or leaner
- Chicken drumstick, skinless
- Chicken leg, skinless
- Chicken, liver
- Chicken patty, plain
- Chicken thigh, skinless
- Chicken breast, oven roasted/rotisserie seasoned, deli-style
- Cornish hen, skinless
- Ground turkey, 90% lean or leaner
- Ground turkey breast
- Turkey breast, skinless
- Turkey, canned in water
- Turkey drumstick skinless
- Turkey leg, skinless
- Turkey, liver
- Turkey, patty, plain
- Turkey thigh, skinless
- Turkey breast, oven roasted/ rotisserie seasoned, deli-style

EGGS

- Eggs
- Egg whites
- Egg yolks
- Eggs, hard-boiled or soft-boiled
- Eggs, scrambled, made without fat
- Liquid egg substitute, made from egg whites

FISH & SHELLFISH

- Abalone
- Alaskan king crab
- Anchovies, canned in water
- Arctic char
- Bluefish
- Branzino
- Butterfish
- Carp
- Catfish
- Caviar
- Clams
- Cod
- Crabmeat, lump
- Crayfish
- Cuttlefish
- Eel
- Fish roe
- Flounder
- Grouper
- Haddock
- Halibut
- Herring
- Lobster
- Mackerel
- Mackerel, canned in water
- Mahi-mahi
- Monkfish
- Mussels
- Octopus
- Orange roughy
- Oysters
- Perch
- Pike
- Pollock
- Pompano
- Salmon
- Sardines, canned in water or sauce
- Sashimi
- Scallops
- Sea bass
- Sea cucumber
- Sea urchin
- Shrimp
- Smelt
- Smoked fish (haddock, salmon, sturgeon, trout, and whitefish)
- Snails
- Snapper
- Sole
- Squid
- Steelhead trout
- Striped bass
- Sturgeon
- Swordfish
- Tilapia
- Trout
- Tuna
- Tuna, canned in water
- Turbot
- Wahoo
- Whitefish

LEAN MEATS

- Beef, arm pot roast, lean, trimmed
- Beef, bottom round, roast or steak, trimmed
- Beef, cube steak, trimmed
- Beef, eye of round roast, lean, trimmed
- Beef, eye of round steak, lean, trimmed
- Beef, filet mignon, lean, trimmed
- Beef, flank steak, lean, trimmed
- Beef, ground 90% lean or leaner
- Beef, Kansas City strip steak, lean, trimmed
- Beef, liver
- Beef, London broil
- Beef, New York strip steak, lean, trimmed
- Beef, rump roast, lean, trimmed
- Beef, strip steak, lean, trimmed
- Beef, tenderloin, lean, trimmed
- Beef, top round roast or steak, trimmed
- Beef, top sirloin steak, lean, trimmed
- Beef, tri-tip roast, lean, trimmed
- Bison, ground, 93% lean
- Bison, lean, trimmed
- Bison, top round steak
- Bison, top sirloin steak
- Elk meat
- Elk, ground, 90% lean (or leaner)
- Goat meat
- Lamb, leg, lean, trimmed
- Lamb, loin, lean, trimmed
- Lamb, sirloin chops, lean, trimmed
- Lamb, tenderloin
- Pork center rib chops, lean, trimmed
- Pork loin chop, lean, trimmed
- Pork sirloin chop, lean, trimmed
- Pork sirloin roast, lean, trimmed
- Pork tenderloin
- Pork, top loin chop, lean, trimmed
- Pork, top loin roast, lean, trimmed
- Rabbit
- Veal cutlet, plain
- Veal loin chop, lean, trimmed
- Veal shank
- Venison
- Venison, ground

OATS

- Oatmeal, plain
- Oatmeal, plain, instant
- Oats, quick-cooking
- Oats, rolled/old fashioned
- Oats, steel cut

CORN & POPCORN

- Corn, canned
- Corn, fresh (sweet, white, or yellow)
- Corn on the cob
- Popcorn, air-popped without oil, butter, or sugar
- Hominy
- Popcorn with salt and/or spice, air-popped without oil, butter, or sugar
- Popping corn (for popping at home)

BEANS, PEAS & LENTILS

- Adzuki beans
- Alfalfa sprouts
- Bean sprouts
- Black beans
- Black-eyed peas
- Cannellini beans
- Chickpeas
- Edamame
- Fava beans
- Great northern beans
- Green peas
- Kidney beans
- Lentils
- Lima beans
- Lupini beans
- Navy beans
- Peas
- Pinto beans
- Refried beans, fat-free, canned
- Soybeans
- Split peas

TOFU & TEMPEH

- Smoked tofu
- Tempeh
- Tofu, firm
- Tofu, silken
- Tofu, soft

YOGURT & COTTAGE CHEESE

- Almond yogurt, plain
- Cottage cheese, plain nonfat
- Greek yogurt, plain nonfat
- Quark, plain, up to 1% fat
- Soy yogurt, plain
- Yogurt, plain nonfat

Conclusion

If there's one thing to take away, it's that eating well doesn't have to be complicated or restrictive. With the ZeroPoint approach, you've been introduced to a way of living that prioritizes balance, enjoyment, and health without the constant burden of tracking every morsel.

Throughout this book, we've explored the ins and outs of the ZeroPoint foods list, showing how incorporating these foods can transform your eating habits. From hearty breakfasts to delectable desserts, you've seen that these meals aren't just about losing weight—they're about nourishing your body and soul.

ZeroPoint foods are everyday foods that you can find in any grocery store, and they're packed with nutrients to keep you full and energized. By focusing on these core ingredients, you've learned to create meals that are satisfying and diverse, without the stress of counting calories or points.

Remember, the ZeroPoint approach isn't just a diet—it's a lifestyle. It's about making smart choices that align with your goals while still enjoying the foods you love. Whether you're preparing a quick weekday dinner or hosting a gathering with friends, the recipes in this book are designed to fit seamlessly into your life.

Let's not forget the practical tips and tools you've gained along the way. From must-have kitchen gadgets to savvy shopping techniques, you've got a toolkit to make cooking enjoyable and efficient. These strategies will help you maintain this lifestyle long after you've tried every recipe in the book.

As you continue your journey, lean on the 30-day meal plan as your guide. It's there to help you maintain focus and integrate these habits into your daily routine. You'll find that with each passing week, making ZeroPoint meals becomes second nature, and you'll enjoy the benefits of a balanced diet without the constant pressure.

The full ZeroPoint foods list and recipe index are at your fingertips whenever you need them. Use these resources to experiment and create your own delicious dishes. There's no limit to the variety and flavors you can explore within the ZeroPoint framework.

It's been a pleasure to guide you through these recipes and share the joys of guilt-free cooking. Remember, this is just the beginning. The habits and skills you've developed here will serve you well as you continue to explore and enjoy food in a way that's both delicious and mindful.

So, here's to a healthier, happier you. Keep experimenting, keep enjoying, and most importantly, keep cooking. You've got all the tools you need to succeed, and I can't wait to see the fantastic meals you'll create. Cheers to a future full of flavor and wellness!

RECIPE INDEX

W

Z

MEASUREMENTS AND CONVERSIONS

VOLUME EQUIVALENTS (DRY)		WEIGHT EQUIVALENTS	
US STANDARD	METRIC (APPROX.)	US STANDARD	METRIC (APPROX.)
1/4 tsp	1.25 ml	1 ounce	28 g
1/2 tsp	2.5 ml	4 ounces	113 g
1 tsp	5 ml	8 ounces	225 g
1/4 cup	60 ml	12 ounces	340 g
1/3 cup	80 ml	One pound (16oz)	455 g
1/2 cup	120 ml		
1 cup	240 ml		

VOLUME EQUIVALENTS (LIQUID)			OVEN TEMPERATURES	
US STANDARD	US OUNCES	METRIC	FAHRENHEIT	CELSIUS (APPROX.)
1 tsp	1/6 oz	5 ml	200° F	93° C
1 tbsp	1/2 oz	15 ml	225° F	107° C
1 fluid ounce	1 oz	30 ml	250° F	120° C
1 cup	8 oz	240 ml	275° F	135° C
1 pint	16 oz	475 ml	300° F	150° C
1 quart	32 oz	950 ml	325° F	165° C
1 gallon	128 oz	3.8 L	350° F	177° C
			375°F	190° C
			400°F	200° C
			425°F	220°C

REFERENCES

1 WeightWatchers. (n.d.-b). Learn about ZeroPoint foods. https://www.weightwatchers.com/uk/how-it-works/zeropoint-foods

2 Cissn, S. P. R. C. C. (2024, May 19). Weight Watchers: Is it Right for You? Verywell Fit. https://www.verywellfit.com/pros-and-cons-of-weight-watchers-3496212

3 WeightWatchers. (2024, December 11). Meet the ZeroPoint® foods. WeightWatchers. https://www.weightwatchers.com/uk/blog/food/full-zeropoint-foods-list